Loving You
From Here

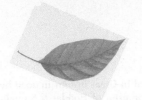

Loving You From Here

STORIES OF GRIEF, HOPE AND GROWTH WHEN A BABY DIES

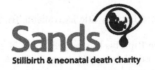

Stillbirth & neonatal death charity

WITH SUSAN CLARK

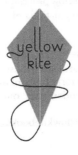

First published in Great Britain in 2020 by Yellow Kite
An imprint of Hodder & Stoughton
An Hachette UK company

1

Sands Charity Registration Number 299679

Sands Scottish Charity Registration Number SC042789

Book title inspired by the song 'I Can Love You From Here'
by Liberty's Mother, Sophie Daniels

A CIP catalogue record for this title is available from the British Library

Trade Paperback ISBN 978 1 529 38275 4
eBook ISBN 978 1 529 38424 6

Typeset in Celeste and Avenir by
Palimpsest Book Production Ltd, Falkirk, Stirlingshire

Printed and bound in Great Britain by Clays Ltd, Elcograf S.p.A.

Hodder & Stoughton policy is to use papers that are natural, renewable
and recyclable products and made from wood grown in sustainable forests.
The logging and manufacturing processes are expected to conform
to the environmental regulations of the country of origin.

Contents

Foreword

By Dr Clea Harmer, Chief Executive of Sands

The death of a baby is a hidden tragedy – both in terms of the intense grief experienced by parents, and also the scale of the problem. Parents and families find themselves plunged into the painful reality of this loss, which is then compounded by the silence surrounding it.

The unique thing about Sands (the leading stillbirth and neonatal death charity in the UK) is that it represents the voice of these bereaved parents and families – a voice which is struggling to make sense of what has just happened, which is finding a way to cope with the grief, and which is trying to make sure that others don't have to go through the same devastating experience. It is this voice of bereaved parents that drives the work that Sands does to reduce the number of babies dying, and to improve care and support for all those affected by the death of a baby. And it is this voice that you will find running through this book which will, in the same way, support all those affected by the death of a baby, including the wider circle of family, friends, neighbours and work colleagues.

Bereaved parents often feel invisible and alone in their grief and being able to reach out and find they are not alone can break through this painful isolation. The support Sands provides is absolutely vital, but we also play a role in making sure that, as a society, we *all* reach out and hold bereaved parents at a time when they most need to be held.

Bereaved parents show enormous generosity – and determination – in making sure that nobody else has to go through what they have been through. They want to know why their baby died, and whether anything could have been done differently; and they want to know that the bereavement care parents receive from hospitals and health professionals is the very best possible and is given to all. We owe it to these parents to make their voices heard – to make sure that their devastating experiences are used to try to make things better for others, and this is what Sands works hard to do.

Key to all of this is breaking the silence and the taboo around baby death. The isolation that parents feel speaks volumes about how society feels unable to talk, or even think, about the tragedy of a baby dying – quite literally struggling to find the words. Raising awareness and making the voice of bereaved parents heard helps to break that silence, and over the years Sands has used different ways to do this. In 2008 our 'Why17?' campaign asked why 17 babies died every day in the UK, and the '#15babiesaday' in 2017 used washing lines with 15 babygros pegged on them to highlight the fact that 15 babies were still dying in the UK every day. In 2018 the number dropped to 14 which is still too high.

As with any other charity, fundraising is key to our work, but fundraising plays a unique role in Sands. For many, raising funds is an integral part of their grief journey – helping to channel the stark and raw feelings, but also helping to do something special in memory of their baby. People run marathons, jump out of planes, climb mountains – but also lovingly bake cakes, knit blankets and host coffee mornings.

Sadly, for many there are very few memories of their baby, and so their fundraising also helps them to make memories and talk about their baby. All our supporters are incredibly special to us, and we treasure what their involvement means to them on every level.

The voice of bereaved parents is so important in so many ways and deserves to be more widely heard. This is at the heart of all that we do at Sands, and of this book, *Loving You From Here*.

'I COULD NOT CRY', BEL MOONEY, *GUARDIAN*, 8 JANUARY 1976

I remembered pushing, breathing through a mouth like the Sahara. Then at 5am I regained consciousness in my small cubicle, staring confusedly at the dim red light they leave burning in the rooms of the sick, wondering what had happened. Needing a bed pan, I groped stiffly for the bell, brain clearing, awareness dawning.

By the time the nurse came I knew – though my hand still felt my stomach to see if he was still there. 'What happened?', I asked. She looked distressed: 'Don't you know? You had your baby and it was a little boy, and he isn't alive.'

For three hours until my husband came, I could not cry. They had taken me into hospital two weeks earlier to rest because of my lack of weight; they had induced the birth three weeks early in a (now I see) desperate attempt to prevent his inevitable death inside me: the night before the labour I rang a friend and said I was convinced my baby would die.

But such is the gap between what the heart hopes and the mind knows, that I could not take in the fate I had predicted. During 16 hours of awful pain made worse by the anxiety, I hoped he would live. I expected him to live. I laboured for his life. Now my husband and I were left to weep in each others' arms – like all parents of stillborn babies devastated by the extent of the love and loss we felt for someone we had never met.

The following days taught me more about the nature of

motherhood, as well as of suffering, than did the birth of my first son, Daniel, now aged two. The gap ached – so much so that one sleepless, tormented night I tiptoed downstairs to get Daniel's teddy bear to take back to bed – the vacancy in the womb had been replaced by an emptiness in my arms and some small thing, anything, was necessary to fill it and they send women to prison for stealing babies.

On the fourth day after the birth-death I awoke to find my breasts full of milk – nature's cruellest irony – ready to feed the baby who was not there. Like a full cow past milking time I cried. And like an animal I could not understand: all the intellectual/feminist debate on the nature of motherhood and the needs of the family dissolved beside the awfulness of the physical loss and need. For nine months I had been prepared for a baby. Without that baby I was still a mother, ready, and cheated. When I cried bitterly three nights in succession that I hated being a woman, hated being married, hated being trapped, I was expressing an awareness more fundamental than that of my role, more an unwilling acceptance of my function.

He was born and died on the Wednesday. On Friday I was discharged from the hospital – the doctors and nurses, though kind and upset, unable (I sensed) to cope. Out of place, amidst waiting pregnant women, and the mewls of the newborn, and postnatally depressed girls staring helplessly into metal cots full of responsibility, had come death, and it was an intrusion.

Some mothers of stillborn babies want to see and hold their dead baby, though I did not. But significantly, it was never suggested. Those who have escaped the experience cannot approach its meaning: that a stillborn child is a real person to the mother (and father, in this case) who bore him/her.

One day at home a friend rang, and I heard my mother say: 'Bel lost her baby.' The euphemism outraged me. For I did not lose him like an umbrella or a lover. He was born and died. To be accurate he was born dead: the ultimate contradiction in terms, so mysterious it defies analysis. When I heard that acquaintances thought I had miscarried I was equally outraged – it seemed important that they should realise the gulf between that sad accident and what we had been through.

That gulf is symbolised most clearly by the requirements of bureaucracy: the fact that my husband had to go, one bleak rainy day, to get a piece of paper from the hospital then go to the Registrar's office and 'give the particulars' – all written out in laborious longhand in the special book for the Stillbirths that are neither Birth nor Death, but both – then return to the hospital with another piece of paper to discuss funerals, prices, whether the ending would be Christian.

Though we did not attend the plain cremation the State requires and provides it was strangely consoling to think of him in his shroud and tiny, named doll's coffin. 'Fitting' is the word: that a life which had begun should be ended with some rudimentary ceremony.

Afterwards, people rang. I wanted to tell the story: to talk about him gave his brief life a meaning, to share the experience with others gave it importance. Morbid it might (superficially) seem, but it was necessary: an exorcism of pain that was also a sharing of love.

Those who have experienced the death of a baby probably feel first (after the tears) the need to blame. In this case, first occurred the possibility that the hospital could have done something. But doctors are not gods, nor is science without its limitations. We assume that the process of pregnancy and birth is without its old perils – though still something like 20 in a thousand babies die. When your baby dies, you look at loaded carry-cots with new wonder, the leap into the world seeming all the more perilous. All that ultra sound equipment, all the knowledge of obstetrics . . . and the doctors, doing all they could, were blameless.

But needing to find a reason, you turn upon yourself. I knew that I had rested as much as I could and eaten well – I had stopped work and cooked nourishing meals of liver and greens I did not want simply to make him grow. But blame lies deeper. The day after his birth-death I raved at my husband like a child: 'I haven't been wicked. I've tried to be good to people. . . I've been a bit wicked but not that wicked.'

The words assumed an area of responsibility far deeper than the physical, more primitive and necessary than sleep or food. I blamed myself in two ways. I felt that I had failed as a woman in that I had not managed to fulfill the sexual function I had assumed (either by conditioning or instinct) as my own. More important, I assumed I had failed as a person: somehow, I had 'gone wrong' and so I was being punished.

By whom? One day a woman who happens to be Catholic visited me at home, and when I explained to her how real that baby seems, and how I am conscious of having borne two sons, she said: 'You realise you are talking in a religious way?' Of course, I did. Though an agnostic I was, for lack of anyone else, blaming God for my son's death.

He was born at midnight though they stopped (unknown to me) listening for his heart at 10.30pm. That was November 26, 1975, his birthday. On the 27th I heard myself asking my husband if our baby had a soul and where had he gone? A friend who had the same experience told me that it made her leave the Catholic Church – she was told that her baby, unbaptised, had gone to Limbo, that terrible empty place they reserve for children who have died without sin, but whose original sin, unredeemed by baptism, has denied them Heaven.

But I discovered, after initial grief and subsequent bitterness and rage, that I do not believe in original sin – just in original goodness. As we shared sorrow my husband consoled me by saying that his own comfort lay in the conviction that his baby died pure – he was conceived, and existed, and died. It was simply a speeding-up of the process we all experience, without the pain, without the regrets, without the hurting of other people, without the sickening consciousness of universal misery, without the disappointments of age. Also, of course, without the moments of joy – but then, he was wanted, cherished, loved, and so in that there is a joy he might have felt. How do we know what the unborn feel?

Without any joy to wipe out the memory I keep remembering the labour and see myself as through the wrong end of a telescope – a creature on a bed, writhing, vomiting, crying, almost unable to hear the physical suffering. Afterwards, longing for my baby to cuddle, I see myself railing at my husband, almost unable to bear the mental anguish. But it is in that 'almost' that the majesty lies. Because we do bear it and we still want to live, all the love and hope and pain and loss, the resilience and acceptance, are all the more precious because of the darkness that surrounds them.

Five days after I came home, I received a letter from a man called George Thatcher, a talented playwright, serving life murder in Gartree for a crime he steadfastly maintains he did not commit and who cannot obtain parole. He had been told about my baby by a mutual acquaintance.

His letter began: 'I'm not going to make you cry because you have shed enough tears. But somewhere along the line there is a joy for you which will surpass all that pain – and only be possible because of it.'

That sentiment – expressed (ironically enough) by someone who after 13 years is still deemed unfit to rejoin society – brought the most comfort, identifying the one thing that, for us, gave our baby's brief existence purpose. There is no divine right to happiness, simply a duty to cope, to understand, and to love. My duty to my first son seems clear and easy; but there is also a duty to that second baby.

I do not wish to 'get over' his loss, nor do I wish to replace him with more children. I simply wish that his life and death should be absorbed into my own: enlarging and deepening in perception.

Introduction

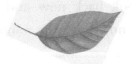

'Those who have escaped the experience cannot approach its meaning: that a stillborn child is a real person to the mother (and father, in this case) who bore him/her.'

From Bel Mooney's 1976 *Guardian* article

The wall of silence that Clea Harmer talks of in the Foreword has been a constant companion to me for almost thirty years following my own loss of three much-wanted babies throughout my thirties, and when I was asked if I would like to work with Sands to create this much-needed book, my first reaction was to run – metaphorically – for the hills and stay in that place of silence.

But something else was tugging around the edges of my conscience and, for want of a better description, it felt like three pairs of tiny hands were asking me to step up and use my professional skills as a writer and journalist to help Sands break the silence and allow other bereaved parents to bravely share not only their painful stories of grief, but also their stories of growth and hope.

I already knew I had grown, slowly but surely, through my own grief, but I did not expect my heart to expand even more by helping these parents to tell their stories and by writing this book. Of course, I look back now and understand it had to expand because I too now have the names and stories of these babies – written, where possible, in their own words by their loving parents – firmly in my heart; and I understand the fire in the belly of the mothers and fathers who find the courage to revisit those painful feelings in order to speak out and who know that, collectively, we need to break this taboo.

When your baby dies, it might feel true that everything else has gone – not just the baby you wanted, but also everything as you once knew it, including and especially your identity and yourself. And so, the task ahead is one of starting anew, which you won't, for a long time, want to do.

The death of a baby is one of the most painful and traumatic things you will ever go through, and when you are a parent whose baby has died you will know all these feelings. What you may not know is what small steps – and they will need to be small – you can take to move forwards without forgetting your baby and what they mean to you. If you are someone trying to support a parent who has come home without their baby – a relative, a friend, a work colleague, a health professional or even a neighbour – it will be a challenge to get up close to the rawness and visceral nature of the pain you are witnessing and not want to run away from it to protect your own sense of some kind of just order in the world.

This book is for anyone whose life has been touched and affected by the death of a baby before, during or after birth. That includes people who have suffered an early or a late miscarriage and those who have had an ectopic pregnancy. Regardless of the stage of the pregnancy or the specific circumstances of a baby dying during or shortly after birth, bereaved parents will share many of the same difficult feelings, all of which we will explore with the help of the stories of other bereaved parents and, using our 40-year-long legacy of working with bereaved parents, we will show you how to manage.

This is also a book that smashes one of our last taboos – the fear of talking about the death of a baby, an event that turns all our preconceived notions of an orderly world with everything in its rightful place upside down. Collectively, and thanks in large part to social media and a generation that has grown up with shared online platforms and fewer inhibitions about talking about 'feelings', we are now having more open conversations about death and bereavement. However, we are still afraid and unsure of what words to use when the death we want to talk about is the death of a baby and when the feelings we are trying to understand and empathise with are those of the shocked and distraught parents.

It is as if we share a collective fear that we might catch those horrible feelings or that they might, in some contagious way, scar our own experiences of the joy of pregnancy and a new baby. It is this fear that has built up a wall of silence around the topic of stillbirth, neonatal deaths and the loss of any wanted pregnancy, and it is this still deeply rooted fear that this book

3

will help us overcome so that we can finally break this alienating taboo which makes an awful experience so much more traumatic than it needs to be.

The Statistics

Every day in the UK, 14 babies will die before, during or shortly after birth. In the UK, a stillbirth is not registered before 24 weeks' gestation (although the government is currently reviewing whether to lower the age of registration to 18 weeks' gestation) so this 2018 figure (the latest available at the time of going to press and one baby less than the previous year) does not include late miscarriages or ectopic pregnancies.

According to UK birth registration figures for 2018, 2958 babies were stillborn. Another 2028 babies died within the first four weeks of being born. That's a combined 4986 stillbirths and neonatal deaths equating to 14 babies dying every day that year. This figure is 345 fewer deaths compared with the previous year (2017) but does not include the death of any baby born before 24 weeks' gestation.

What these figures mean in terms of human heartache is that roughly every two hours, a mother, a father and the family who love them and were waiting to love the new baby, are catapulted to a deep, dark place, with many never getting a satisfactory answer to the question that will haunt them for the rest of their lives: why?

This is the biggest question bereaved parents want the answer to. However, sadly, most of us won't get any kind of answer, let alone one that would allow us to make our peace with the death of our babies before, during or shortly after birth. So it's no surprise that the three core tenets underpinning the work of Sands are:

1 Saving babies' lives.
2 Ensuring all parents receive excellent bereavement care.
3 Providing bereavement support for all those who need it after the death of a baby.

> The UK government says that it now aims to halve the rates of stillbirths and neonatal deaths by 2025, with an interim ambition to achieve a 20 per cent reduction in those rates by 2020. The ambition includes similar reductions in maternal mortality and serious brain injuries in babies during or soon after birth, and a 25 per cent reduction in the pre-term birth rate from the current 8 per cent to 6 per cent by 2025.

The fact is that, according to the Royal College of Obstetricians and Gynaecologists, the outcome for three quarters of babies who died at the end of pregnancy might have been different with different care. The UK government itself reported recently that an estimated 600 stillbirths could be avoided annually if all maternity units adopted national best practice, and Sands has long been campaigning and lobbying for the improvements in maternity care that will see fewer babies dying and meet that ambitious goal of a 50 per cent reduction in stillbirths and neonatal deaths by 2025.

Meanwhile, parents, like this bereaved mother whose second baby, Xanthe, was stillborn, are left reeling by the lack of an explanation as to why their baby died. And for some bereaved parents, worse than not getting any explanation over why their baby died is any suggestion that lifestyle choices may somehow be to blame:

'I have read many things about associations between stillbirth and socio-economic deprivation; stillbirth and caffeine consumption; stillbirth and alcohol consumption; stillbirth and previous caesarean birth. None of these things apply in our situation.

'I am sure there are many people who have had a stillborn baby who, like us, find that the scant research there has been does not apply to them either. The correlations/links that have been addressed generally turn the blame to the mother, something which is grossly unfair. I have read also that many unexplained stillborn babies show poor foetal growth; again, this was not the case with our daughter. It seems outrageous that no one has any idea what caused our daughter to die.'

According to the World Health Organization (WHO), which recommends a definition of stillbirth as being the birth of a baby born with no signs of life at or after 28 weeks' gestation, the causes of stillbirth worldwide include:

- childbirth complications
- post-term pregnancy
- maternal infections in pregnancy
- maternal disorders (especially hypertension, obesity and diabetes)
- foetal growth restriction
- congenital abnormalities

And again, according to WHO, almost half of all stillbirths, globally, happen during labour and the majority are preventable. *Preventable.*

The Story of Sands

The story of Sands started 42 years ago when two bereaved mothers, journalist Bel Mooney and Hazelanne Lewis, decided, after discovering there was zero support for them or any other bereaved parent following the death of their babies, something had to be done.

Bel's article about the death of her baby boy had been published in the *Guardian* newspaper on 8 January 1976, and blew the lid off a subject so secretive not only did nobody ever talk about it, most mothers never even knew what had happened to the baby they had given birth to and who had died. (Bel Mooney's original article is reproduced in full on pages x–xv.)

Hazelanne, whose baby son had also died the year before, contacted Bel after reading her article and the rest, as they say, is history . . .

At that time – the mid-1970s – in the UK, most parents were

7

not allowed to see, hold or have a funeral for their babies. No photographs were taken, and they could not put their baby's name on the stillbirth registration certificate. And, even today, Sands staff, the charity's support groups and volunteers get calls from elderly mothers of stillborn babies asking whether Sands can help them find out what happened to their baby. (Happily, there are times when the charity can track back and locate a baby's grave and give those still-grieving mothers the closure they are seeking.)

The first Sands newsletter went out in 1980, and after three years of meetings with the UK Charity Commission, in 1981 Bel and Hazelanne registered the Stillbirth and Perinatal Death Association (SPDA) as a charity. That name changed to Sands (Stillbirth and Neonatal Death Society) in 1984, and in 1987 the familiar Sands teardrop logo was introduced.

The new charity set up a helpline in 1985 and published a booklet called 'Saying goodbye to your baby'. In 1991 the first guidelines for professionals were published, and in 1992 the definition of stillbirth was reduced from 28 weeks (still the current WHO recommendation) to 24 weeks in the UK, thanks to the Sands Act after that bill received royal assent.

Leap forwards almost a quarter of a century and, in 2016, the All-Party Parliamentary Group (APPG) on Baby Loss was formed bringing together MPs and peers to improve care for bereaved parents and raise the issues around baby death within Parliament.

Things were starting to shift, slowly but surely.

In 2018, Sands built further on the foundations of its now long history of groundbreaking awareness and bereavement care improvement initiatives by collaborating in the launch of the Perinatal Mortality Review Tool (PMRT). This not only supports hospitals in conducting high-quality reviews after a baby has died – so that lessons learned from those reviews can be used to improve future care – but, just as importantly, puts bereaved parents at the very heart of the review by taking into account their perspectives of the care they received when their baby died and, by doing so, helps more parents understand why that happened.

At the heart of the story of Sands, underpinning every new campaign and initiative, lies the same hope that has shaped this book, namely that one day far fewer bereaved parents will be crying over the death of their baby, that the number of babies dying will have fallen and, when it does happen, parents will get the answers they need and feel heard by everyone involved.

This book is not just for bereaved parents, but for all those whose lives are impacted when a baby dies, at whatever age or gestation. It is a book for the grieving parents and upset medical professionals, and it is also for friends and relatives and neighbours and work colleagues and anyone else who knows a baby has died but who may not know what to say and be so scared of saying 'the wrong thing' that they end up saying nothing at all.

Many families have shared the intimate details and pain of their stories throughout this book, all shared in the hope that they may say or reveal something in the telling and exploration of their journey to a new normal that will help and inspire other bereaved parents and those supporting them. The stories and personal experiences show just one individual viewpoint and of course different cultures, and different people, will grieve and move on in different ways. Alongside these stories, there is practical guidance and advice that may help families find their new normal after a baby has died.

Liberty's Legacy

The title of this book – *Loving You From Here* – was inspired by the song 'I Can Love You From Here', written by Liberty's mother, singer/songwriter Sophie Alagna (professional name Sophie Daniels) who is now mum to Cosmo, six, and Rocco, five, and wife to Alessandro. She is also – very actively – mum to her first-born daughter, Liberty, who died in January 2011, 36 weeks into the pregnancy. On the day before she was stillborn, doctors failed to spot Sophie's placenta had died.

Here are the lyrics (the song is available to stream or download, and for more information go to www.libertysmother.com):

I CAN LOVE YOU FROM HERE
By Liberty's mother

I know that love will come and go
That there's much less sun than rain
But, for me, there's little left to learn
If I can't hold you again

I try to look ahead but there's nothing left to see
But, it doesn't matter anymore, if you're next to me

(Chorus)

'Cause I can love you from here
Hold that love in my heart
I can find a way to give that love a life, now we're apart

Introduction

I don't know why you're gone
But the rest is so clear
All I need is to love you
And I can love you from here

I know it's better to love and lose it all
Than to never even try
Still it seems so hard, to come and break my heart
And then leave me with no reason why

Why we're not together, I'll never understand
But I don't need to be with you, to love you like I
    planned

(Chorus)

No matter how I ask, you're never coming back
But this love is never going to die away

(Chorus)

© *Sophie Daniels, March 2011*

Sophie says she often thinks being Liberty's mum is the most important part of her identity and her song, which will touch the heart of anyone who is mourning the loss of someone they love, is particularly potent for those of us who have dead babies in our hearts and minds with whom we never got to make years of memories.

It's an idea that resonates with all the bereaved parents who

11

have heard it and not least because it's such a positive and active affirmation of feelings that will persist lifelong.

I *can* love you from here . . . I *am* loving you from here . . .

Here is what Sophie says about the song she wrote just 10 weeks after her beloved daughter died:

'I Can Love You From Here' explores the idea of a 'continuous bond'. It's an expression of the limitless love that I have for my child which will always continue, even though Liberty is gone.

We parents of babies who are gone need to retain our bond with them and it is a healthy and positive thing. We need to use their names and to continue to speak of them and celebrate their lives, however brief. Because they were here and they were real, and they were and always will be our children.

When I wrote the song, I felt a real sense of relief – like I had cracked some code. I realised that I can always love her and that I must speak her name every chance I get, even though others may feel confronted by the fact of life and death. Her life and death is a reality, and my love and respect for my child will always be more important than any stranger's, or indeed friend's, discomfort when coming into this topic.

Over time, I have come to realise that Liberty's legacy is so very many things. It's everything she has taught me. It's the strength and love that she has embedded into this family of five. It is the song that I wrote for her and, I hope, the love that the song will spread wherever it goes.

The song is about love's triumph over grief. Because grief is incredibly hard, but in the end, love is stronger, and the love that Liberty left behind has made us all strong. It is a strength filled with and fuelled by love.

I hope that all parents who lose their children can find a way to feel the same.

What Sophie is talking about is a new normal and this book, just like her song, shows that no matter how devastated newly bereaved parents feel, there is a new normal waiting for them and one that is built on the values of hope and love.

Writing the book has been a slow and painstaking process because grief is so complex. The subject, to take a quote from later in the book, is 'too big, too painful' and yet *Loving You From Here* (thanks to all those who have contributed) rises to that challenge of breaking the silence surrounding baby death, of supporting bereaved parents and those who are trying to support them, and finally smashing one of our last great taboos.

> **This book was written during the COVID-19 pandemic. In finding their new normal, Sands put a lot of their support – including support group meetings – online. For the latest information on how Sands can support you, please visit their website www.sands.org.uk/ support-you**

CHAPTER 1

When Your Baby Dies

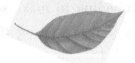

'I am depressed, saddened, hurt, empty, guilty and lonely. I cry every day. I will mourn him forever.'

A bereaved mother from the 2018 *Lancet* series on stillbirth

When your baby dies, so does a part of you. The person who, for years, looked back at you from the mirror is gone for good. Shattered into a thousand tiny shards, each one waiting to cut, pierce and wound, no matter how carefully you, or those who love you, try to pick them up to put you back together.

In so many ways, finding your way through this shattering loss will be a lifelong challenge. The first hurdle being the fact that you don't want to be a different you. You don't want to put together a new version to face the world or even stay away from it; you want the old you and what you want back, more than anything and with an anguished yearning so intense you don't know how you will survive that pain, let alone function normally, is the baby who has just died.

This then is the hidden terrain – a kind of scrubby, murky hinterland – from which you will have to find your way back to the world. It's a harsh and usually lonely place. There may be two of you in it, since it takes two to make a baby, but at first, you likely won't be able to see, let alone support, each other. There's just too much pain and sorrow.

There are others struggling to make sense of finding themselves here too; other parents facing the same challenge of navigating this unmapped territory, but their presence will be and feel as shadowy as your own because dead babies is not something anyone knows how to talk about.

There are no bells or birds in this place where you find yourself when your baby first dies. No baby showers, birthday celebrations, nursery rhymes or daydreams. The silence is oppressive and suffocating and the sun does not shine. If hope, of any kind, is still in the mix, it's not here but somewhere else that you cannot reach or even imagine.

This feeling of hopelessness is normal when your baby has just died. You are still in shock. But, over time, as with all bereavement, the shock will lessen, and you will learn to manage your grief. Happily, the stories in this book – although painful to read – show that, with time and with the courage to keep going, you will find your way back to hope.

Some days you might take a tiny step forwards, only to find yourself waking up the next day full of all the grief and fury and hopelessness you thought had gone. You are making progress, each and every day, although it may not feel like it. But if you can trust in the stories of grief, hope and growth that those who have gone before you are sharing in this book then you can start to believe it will be the same for you.

Right now though, when your baby has just died, you may not yet feel ready to let go of any part of the pain you are in. You may feel scared that if you do, you might forget your baby. Then you would no longer feel like any kind of a parent, not even a bad one who couldn't launch their baby into life. You might feel nothing, which would be worse than feeling annihilated by your loss.

The word 'loss' will make you wince each time you hear it; 'I'm sorry you lost your baby. Let me know if there is anything I/we can do.'

You want to scream: 'I didn't lose my baby. My baby was snatched away from me. I know exactly where my baby is. I'm not such a bad parent I would lose my child.'

Of course, you do no such thing. That deathly thicket of silence is there for a reason, mainly to protect other people, so you probably just say 'thank you' and slip back into exile in the fortress to eye up the pile of shattered glass that was once you.

You are lonely but not alone in the fortress. You have an uninvited roommate whom nobody else wants to live with either: Grief. It's the only thing in this place which is not shadowy. Rather, a rambunctious character who shows up at all the wrong times, grabs hold of you at the very moment you glimpse a little respite – a little hope – and chucks you against the wall of your shared cell (grief can be a very violent and antisocial entity) to get your attention. And having got it, stamps on you for fun just to make sure you know who is boss in this relationship.

Hope is your destination, and you will find it again, but you will need the support of those who love you as well as those who have already passed this way before you. And once you start to shape a new normal – one that is built on the enduring bond we will show you how to form with your baby who died – you will wake up one morning and realise that, although you are no longer the same person, you are actually much more of a person. You have more compassion, you have a bigger heart; and you may even have a strong desire to give something back.

All these changes are changes that have happened because your baby died. There are so many stories here of bereaved parents who once, perhaps just as you feel now, struggled to see any way out of the pain but who slowly, and with the help of others, learned to grieve healthily and move on without losing sight of the love for their baby who died. They can now talk honestly about what happened and how it felt; they have found ways to still celebrate their baby's life and place in their family; and many, as you will discover through the chapters of this book, have even gone on to help other families whose baby has just died.

Remember as you read on, whether you are a newly bereaved parent or someone trying to love and care for someone who is, everyone who has shared their story here has lived through all of the very difficult and painful feelings you are going through right now. And all have survived.

They all found hope. Hope found them.

The Silence

After the death of their baby, many bereaved parents go straight to the kind of bleak and lonely hinterland we have just described. They don't want to. Society wants them to. Or maybe, more truthfully, it's a mutual unspoken pact. You agree to disappear while going through the motions of your resumed (minus baby) life and society nods its approval because showing up with all your unresolved feelings of grief and anger and injustice and rage and jealousy and misery does not make for a very charming guest. No, thank you!

We have a collective respect for grief, and not least because we will all experience some version of it. We send cards, we send flowers. My house looked like a florists when my first baby died and all I really wanted to do was throw them out, smash the vases and go back to the pregnant me who still had her baby.

As those flowers – just like my tiny baby had – died, and as the withered blooms were discarded into the waste bin, a deathly hush settled over the household with nobody able to find the words – right or wrong ones – to build a bridge, even a wobbly one, back to the outside world which I felt no longer had a space for me or my missing baby.

At the hospital, we had been 'Mum' and 'baby' until things started to go wrong, when we instantly became 'the patient' and 'the foetus'. This is something that many bereaved parents experience – the sudden flip into medical speak – and, while it can feel hurtful, it isn't meant to be, so this is one of the first inadvertent 'hurts' you may want to just forgive.

Induction was started (they thought I had an infection which had caused my waters to break prematurely, although that turned out to be wrong) and the clock slowed to a different dragging version of time as we waited – the baby's dad and me, and a very frightened young midwife – for something nobody wanted to happen and nobody knew how to stop.

I will spare you the detail of what happened next. Or maybe, even with the passage of three decades since the death of that

19

first baby, I will spare myself. I'm not sure I even remember, except for the very worst bits, but I do recall feeling terrified when it was all over and I was asked if I would like to go and see my dead child.

I did not. I knew that if I went to see him it would make it real: he really would be dead and gone.

Someone, I don't remember who, told my husband it would help us both to say goodbye to him, so he agreed. I thought that took great courage on his part; a courage it took me the rest of that day, a Saturday, to find.

When I saw the not-yet-a-proper-baby I had delivered, I felt a rush of guilt and failure mixed with a sweet tenderness. I was afraid to touch his tiny fingers and afraid that if I let myself really feel what his death meant to me I would break into a thousand pieces.

I did everything I could to block out those unbearable feelings of loss, and looking back now through the lens of time and seeing how I found myself catapulted to the hinterland, I realise I was guilty of the pact of silence and of not knowing how to speak about something that had switched, in a heartbeat, from joyful and innocent – pregnancy and those first tentative imaginings of parenthood – to a nightmare experience that I thought I must have deserved (why else would it have happened?) and would have to bury to survive.

What we did bury was that tiny human-no-longer-being. My best friend and her husband came with us. Which was very brave. And we never spoke of it again until 30 years later when I was talking about writing this book and they reminded me we had had a funeral.

How could I have forgotten?

It is normal to block and suppress feelings that feel unbearable, but it is healthier, in the long run, to experience them, especially when you can do that with the support of others who have had a similar experience or who work with bereaved parents and so have been trained to hold your hand through these first awful months of shock and grief.

You may feel alone in these first days and weeks of coming home from hospital without your baby, but you are not alone. There is support and help for you – much of it in place thanks to those who have gone before over the last 40-plus years and who have shared their experiences with other parents and with Sands – and it is available to you as soon as you are ready to ask for it and for as long as you need it.

You can contact the Sands helpline to talk to an advisor, you can share your story with the online community of bereaved parents, you can download the Bereavement Support app, you can join your local Sands support group or you can ask to be put in touch with a Sands Befriender – another bereaved parent trained specifically to hold your hand through the shock of your loss and the subsequent grief.

Everybody grieves differently so trust your own internal voices which will tell you what you need. What you need will be what is right for you.

Left Alone

Every parent whose baby has died talks of feeling and finding themselves utterly alone with their grief. Too many say they leave hospital after the shock and the trauma with nothing else;

no follow-ups and no advice on what to do next to navigate the terrible onslaught of grief that has rained down on them.

This book aims to step into that empty space and be that supportive first step for newly bereaved parents and those trying to look out for them, all of whom now find themselves in a strange new world and not one anyone would choose to visit.

Funeral directors talk about a certain type of grief etched on the faces of bereaved parents – a withdrawing into themselves, especially the mothers, who can't understand what has just happened and who, numb with shock, may be feeling nothing at all.

It doesn't help that because we all grieve differently, the other parent, if this is a shared experience, will be struggling with their own feelings and may be in a different kind of pain and in a different stage of grief. You may feel exhausted not only by the emotional demands of your grief but by the physical shock of no longer being pregnant but not having your baby with you, and by all the decisions you are being asked to make about the practicalities of what happens after a baby dies or a pregnancy suddenly ends.

This is where support – whether you make a call to the Sands helpline, find your answers in this book or seek out a local support group – matters most. You don't have to go through all this on your own.

CHAPTER 2

What Happens Now?

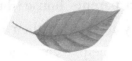

*'The next morning, we got up and travelled back to
Dumfries in order to have our baby. We arrived at
8am and I was put on the drip and by 5.27pm,
baby Abby was born. All I remember from 5.27pm
on 7 June onwards is the silence. No one spoke after
she was born. Robert and I just cried. There was no
baby cry though. There was no conversation from
the midwife because what was there to be said?
There was just silence . . .'*

Bereaved mum

It's the middle of the night, Christmas Eve, 2015, and a young,
bereaved mother, unable to sleep, is alone at the computer
entering a heartbreaking search following the harrowing death
of her baby boy the week before.

'What do you do when your baby dies in Cambridge?' is her question.

Kym Field was just 25 when she sat in despair at the computer to ask that heart-rending question. Baby Alfie had died after labour failed to kick in two days after Kym's waters first broke, and so while the rest of the world was celebrating Christmas and preparing for the big day, Kym and her husband, Mark, had to think about funeral directors and headstones.

Everyone else in her parents' house (the couple could not face returning to an empty nursery at their own home) was asleep and, as she searched for help, Kym, who was too tormented by grief to sleep, believed this painful 'space' was where she was destined to now spend the rest of her life. In fact, she could not even begin to imagine a life without the baby she had not come home with.

ALFIE: BORN 19 DECEMBER 2015

Following a straightforward and enjoyable pregnancy, I was admitted to hospital at around midnight on Friday 18 December 2015 for induction of labour. My waters had broken on the Wednesday and baby was quite clearly staying put for as long as possible!

After a seemingly pretty uneventful labour which I got through using breathing techniques, squeezing pretty much anyone's hand I could get hold of and a little gas and air (OK – a lot of gas and air!), our baby was born.

Immediately the room filled with people and my husband was pushed to one side of the room. I remember the utter silence in the room. 'Not all babies cry as soon as they are born,' I reassured myself. I was desperate to know whether we had a boy or a girl and eventually they told us we had a baby boy and asked if we had chosen a name. I told them he was to be called Alfie.

Alfie was briefly shown to us and whisked off. We were told he had gone to NICU, but details were sketchy. I was taken off for stitches and so my husband was left alone in the delivery room wondering what on earth had just taken place in front of him.

I remember being wheeled past all the new mums and their babies and assuming ours would be cuddled up to my husband when I got back. But he wasn't. A nurse from NICU came to talk to us but all I remember was being told we had a 'very poorly boy'.

When we visited Alfie for the first time, he was perfect in every way despite being covered in wires and beeping machines. We saw past all that. He was our perfect boy.

We were advised to arrange a christening for him. He was just 12 hours old. I remember looking around at the family and friends who had gathered and feeling upset that they were all crying. I had just given birth to a perfect baby in time for Christmas and they were standing around crying. They didn't have the mist of post-birth euphoria like I did. I really believed we would all be home in time for Christmas just like we had planned.

The next day our world crumbled. We were told Alfie had a severe brain injury and would not survive. Words can never describe how we felt in that moment. Even now when I say those words or think about that moment, I feel like I can't breathe.

Alfie died peacefully aged 36 hours old, surrounded by family. We spent the night on the antenatal ward where we had to endure the sounds of babies crying and women in labour, which was torturous; and the next day we were just sent on our merry way to navigate this new life for ourselves.

Almost six months later the hospital trust admitted Alfie's injuries were caused by a misinterpretation of his CTG (heart monitor) trace during my labour.

We are so grateful we had great family support because without it I'm not sure we could have got through it. I think it's so important for health professionals to know you can't fix us or the situation when a baby has died. We just need to be shown the care and compassion any woman should be given after they have given birth. All I wanted for the time I was in hospital was for someone to hold my hand and show us a little bit of empathy.

Thinking back to that night when she was at the computer, Kym says: 'I honestly didn't know what to do. I did that Google search in desperation. I was just looking for someone to help us.'

Kym and Mark are now parents to second son, Barnaby, three, and a little girl, D'Arcy, who is one. 'Life almost four years on is certainly not the one we had planned. Days are still filled with anxiety, tears and a huge hole in our lives that can never be replaced. The pain and loss of Alfie never gets any less or easier to deal with – time just makes it easier to carry the immense weight,' says Kym.

By the time of the inquest into Alfie's death, Kym says she and

Mark understood that he died as a result of 'a collection of errors' by the medical staff, including a misinterpretation of the trace monitoring his heart rate through the labour. The fact the midwife had to call four times for a doctor's assessment during the birth suggested, says Kim, that she knew something was not right but had allowed herself to be overruled by the attending doctors.

Understanding What Happened

If, like Alfie, a baby dies after birth and the cause of death is not clear then the doctor looking after you and your baby must, by law, refer the case to a coroner if you are in England, Wales and Northern Ireland, or to a procurator fiscal if you live in Scotland. The coroner may decide to take no further action and refer the baby's death to the registrar, or the coroner may order an inquest (see page 30) to try to determine what went wrong.

A POST-MORTEM

A post-mortem is a clinical investigation to help understand any factors that might have contributed to your baby's death. When a baby is stillborn or dies after birth, parents are offered a post-mortem and are given information to help them decide whether it is right for them and their baby. Usually, it is a senior health professional who will talk with you about the option of having a post-mortem examination.

A post-mortem will usually provide the most useful information if carried out within a few days of the baby's death. If you need to hold the funeral within 24 or 48 hours, you need to tell the staff at the hospital as they may be able to arrange a post-mortem within this time. Sometimes babies need to be transported to specialist centres in other hospitals where post-mortems can be carried out.

If a post-mortem is needed or agreed on, you will usually have the opportunity to spend time with your baby in hospital or to take them home. The hospital staff will give you advice on how to keep your baby cool so that their condition does not deteriorate. You may be able to borrow a 'cold cot' or unit from the hospital, or a nearby children's hospice, to take home with you.

The thought of a post-mortem can be very frightening for bereaved parents who don't want their baby to come to any harm, but rest assured, throughout this process your baby will be well looked after and treated with respect. You can see and spend time with your baby until it is time for the post-mortem. When your baby is taken away for the examination, you can ask that comforting keepsakes such as soft toys and blankets go with him or her. You can also, if you wish, see your baby again after the post-mortem, although most parents will choose to say goodbye beforehand.

What can a post-mortem tell you?

A post-mortem examination of your baby and of the placenta (afterbirth) may help to find out exactly why your baby died, but even if it cannot do that, it may help by ruling out what didn't cause the death. Here are a few examples of why a post-mortem might be useful:

- It can confirm or change an existing diagnosis.
- It may identify conditions that have not been diagnosed previously.
- It can exclude some common causes of death, such as medical problems with your baby, infections or growth restrictions.
- It may tell you the gender of the baby.
- It can help assess the chances of problems recurring in a future pregnancy.
- It can help provide information about a genetic condition.
- If you already know the immediate cause of your baby's death, a post-mortem may be able to confirm this or may highlight additional problems that might be useful for you to know for a possible future pregnancy.

Everyone recognises that a post-mortem, whether the parents have chosen one or not, is a very difficult decision and one that has to be made when parents are still reeling from the shock of their baby's death. A bereaved mother may feel she is still recovering from the physical experience of the labour and, if still affected by any medications she has taken, simply cannot think clearly. As we have seen, there are good reasons to ask for a post-mortem but you will need help making that decision, so don't feel rushed into it and take the time to speak with family and your hospital advisors so you will feel your voice was heard and you made the right decision for you and your family.

Unless ordered by the coroner, a post-mortem cannot take place without your consent and, even when you have given consent, you can change your mind and withdraw it. If you are struggling to make this decision and in any doubt about giving your consent, ask the hospital how much time you have to change your mind if you do give consent.

It takes a long time for the results of a post-mortem to come through and, unfortunately, often it will not find answers. The consultant should contact you to talk you through the results.

AN INQUEST

When a baby dies as a newborn the hospital must, by law, inform the coroner (or procurator fiscal in Scotland). It is their job then to ascertain where and when the baby died. They can establish the cause of death and determine whether it is thought to be 'unnatural'. If the coroner is concerned about the circumstances of the baby's death being suspicious, they will open an investigation and then possibly an inquest. The coroner may then write a report about any specific concerns.

If, like baby Alfie's parents, you face the prospect of an inquest after your baby has died, the following information will be helpful in preparing for that ordeal. It has been compiled to help you understand the process of a coroner's inquest and make you aware of some of the rights you have.

There are four main objectives of the inquest (who, when, where and how):

1 To establish *who* has died.
2 To establish *when* your baby died.
3 To establish *where* your baby died.
4 To establish *how* your baby died – meaning the medical cause of the death of your baby, and how this happened.

It is important to note that the purpose of the inquest is not to blame or accuse anyone or their actions, it is to establish the facts. That said, the coroner should be putting you, as the family, at the heart of the inquest process.

Once the coroner starts the hearing, the first person to give evidence will usually be the pathologist who will talk about the medical causes of your baby's death. It is not the role of the pathologist to examine all the details that led to the death – that is the purpose of the inquest.

After the pathologist has given their evidence, the coroner will then call on those witnesses he or she believes can give evidence that will allow them to establish the events that led to the death. The coroner can call upon the nurses and doctors involved in the care of your baby to give evidence of what happened and to help them establish the facts that led to the death of your baby. The coroner may also call upon a representative from the hospital trust to be questioned.

The coroner won't always question a witness (whether a family member, a doctor or anyone else) or ask them to give evidence in person; if someone's evidence is not controversial and unlikely to be challenged it can be submitted as a written statement instead. And while questions (provided they fall within the scope of the enquiry) can be asked of all witnesses, the witnesses cannot be cross-examined as if on trial in a criminal court.

Key information for parents*

- The coroner will ask for a spokesperson for the family. You may wish to be the spokesperson, or you may want to nominate another family member; you are perfectly within your rights to do this. Or you can engage a lawyer to represent you and ask questions on your behalf.
- Every witness giving evidence in person at the inquest hearing (including you if you are asked to give evidence) will be asked to either swear an oath on a Bible (or whichever holy book you may choose according to your faith) or, if you prefer, you will be asked to give an affirmation – a non-religious version of an oath.
- It is worth writing a list of questions that you want answering at the inquest in advance to submit to the coroner to ensure they are answered. You should send this document in to the coroner at the earliest opportunity.
- If you have any concerns over the inquest before it starts, then you should write to the coroner. The coroner should be able to answer and manage any concerns as part of keeping you at the heart of the inquest.
- If it is identified that disciplinary measures have been taken at a hospital against an individual, the coroner has no power to reveal those issues. These might only be revealed at a hearing by the GMC (General Medical Council) or the Nursing and Midwifery Council which is separate to the inquest.
- In the instance of a criminal case pending over the death,

---

* Reproduced with grateful thanks from the Sands Bristol support group. Further information and support can be found at www.avma.org.uk.

the coroner will not be able to hold the inquest until the criminal case is over. Once the case is over, depending on the outcome, the coroner may only be able to agree/abide by the criminal case result and a full inquest may not take place.

- Currently legal aid is not generally available to parents for an inquest into the death of a baby unless there are 'exceptional circumstances', but this is very rare. So, unless you can find a solicitor who is able to supply their services free of charge, you will be liable for your own legal costs. If there is a claim being considered, sometimes the costs of having a lawyer at the inquest can be covered but usually not all the costs – you would need to discuss this with your lawyer.
- If you are considering a claim, contact a specialist lawyer (who deals with inquests and, for example, clinical negligence claims) at the earliest possible opportunity.
- There is no right of appeal over the coroner's conclusions. The conclusion can only be reviewed by a Judicial Review if there is evidence/a suggestion that the way the inquest has been managed, or the conclusion of the coroner, is wholly unreasonable.

REVIEWS AND INVESTIGATIONS

Reviews are another important way of trying to understand why your baby died and identify any learning for the future. What is being reviewed is the care that both you as the mother and your baby received; and this includes the care during pregnancy, during labour and when a baby died after birth. This is part of established and standard NHS practice and all baby deaths should be reviewed.

There are different types of reviews and the one you will have will depend on the specific circumstances of your baby's death and whether serious concerns about the care you and your baby received have been raised.

1 The hospital review: known as the Perinatal Mortality Review Tool (PMRT) in England, Wales and Scotland, this is a review of care that should be carried out for all babies who die after 22 weeks' gestation.
2 NHS Serious Incident Investigation (SII): this review will only happen if it is thought something may have gone wrong with the quality of NHS care.
3 In England, there may be a Healthcare Safety Investigation Branch (HSIB) investigation for babies born at 37 weeks or later.
4 The coroner (England) or procurator fiscal (Scotland) can order an inquest where there are serious concerns about the circumstances of the death.

Hospital reviews

The death of a baby before or shortly after birth should always be reviewed by the hospital to understand what happened. This review is designed to support you and other members of your family to understand why your baby died. It could also help to prevent other babies from dying of the same cause.

In the weeks after your baby died, the hospital will hold a review meeting. The review meeting will:

- Try to understand what happened and why your baby died.
- Answer any questions or concerns you may have.
- Look at medical records and test results, including a post-mortem if you have consented to one.
- Talk to staff involved.
- Look at guidance and policies.

The review may also provide the hospital with information that it needs to change the way that staff work. It could also reveal that the care provided was not at fault, but there were other contributory factors.

Your thoughts, feelings and questions are important and need to be considered in this review. Before you leave hospital, staff should inform you about the review process and ask you if you would like to share your experience or ask any questions about your care. To support you in doing this, the hospital should provide you with a key review contact. Your key review contact will:

- Call you within 10 days of your going home to inform you again about the review process.
- Ask if you would like to ask any questions or share your concerns with the review team.
- Give you choices about how you might contribute to the review, either in person, online or via telephone or email.

It can take many weeks to gather all the information required for a review process. This can feel like a very long time to wait for answers and so you can ask your key review contact to arrange a meeting with a consultant before the review itself takes place. Be aware though, the hospital may not yet have any further information at the time of that meeting about why your baby died.

Once the review report has been completed, a consultant can discuss the findings with you. The hospital can also send you the review report by post or email if you prefer. For more information about the PMRT hospital review process, go to: www. npeu.ox.ac.uk/pmrt/information-for-bereaved-parents

NHS Serious Incident Investigations (SII)

If something has gone wrong that may have caused your baby's death, an urgent investigation called an NHS Serious Incident Investigation (SII) will start. This is so that the NHS can be open and honest with families about any mistakes and learn lessons that could prevent future harm or deaths. The NHS should take the views of families into account when deciding whether or not an SII is needed.

The baby deaths in maternity and neonatal care that trigger an SII will usually include a death where the mother arrived in labour close to her due date but the baby subsequently and unexpectedly died either during labour, at birth or shortly after.

Healthcare Safety Investigation Branch (HSIB) investigations

In England, if your baby died at term (37 weeks or more) due to an unexpected event, it may be investigated by the Healthcare Safety Investigation Branch (HSIB). Like an NHS SII, it will carry out an investigation if your baby died during or after delivery because something went wrong in labour. The difference between an NHS SII and an HSIB review is that HSIB investigations are not run by staff from the trust where the baby was born or died. An NHS hospital review will still be carried out even if an HSIB investigation is also being done, but any hospital review will not conclude its findings until the HSIB has finalised its report. For more information about this independent review process, see: www.hsib.org.uk/maternity

If You Choose to Have a Funeral

I thought it would be revealing to talk with someone who is no stranger to grief and who has first-hand experience of the additional layers of challenge the death of a baby brings to the parents, and to those trying to support them, which is how I found myself sitting down with a funeral director, and walking out again feeling deeply moved not only by his insights but by what I can only describe as his professional feelings of 'tenderness' towards all parents whose baby has died. Depending on your cultural and personal beliefs you may or may not feel that a funeral is important for your baby. Funerals can be arranged by the hospital on your behalf, or you may like to create a secular or religious ceremony/activity of your own.

'In death, life is changed, not ended.'
From the Catholic Church funeral eulogy

Like his father and grandfather before him, Clive Wakely is a funeral director and head of a family business based in the south-west of England. After more than 40 years in the trade, he is more than used to being 'the person nobody wants to see', especially at the usually sudden and always traumatic ending of a wanted pregnancy. Handling the arrangements for the bereaved family of a baby who has died requires a 'heightened sensitivity' to the nature of their loss, he says, and brings out feelings of tenderness both towards the child and their grieving parents.

When a family has had the expectation of a child and then it's taken from them when they come into contact with us, we have to manage the loss of what their hopes were, as well as the death of their baby.

They will have had an idea of what the child would be bringing to their family and, often, when it is their first baby that has died, that can be the most difficult because people will say, 'Don't worry, you're still young, you can try again.' But that's taking them down a road they shouldn't be thinking about yet. They should be thinking about dealing with the grief of losing someone.

If the baby has gone full-term and the mother has had to give birth knowing her baby has already died, I don't think we can fully understand what that mother has had to go through. It is very difficult. There's often a feeling that they don't feel worthy and a real sense that they have failed.

For us, there is a marked difference in dealing with people asking for our services when someone has died having lived a life and having contributed to the lives of those around them and dealing with those asking for a service for a baby whom they had hoped would live a life. There is a lot more sensitivity required because, often, the parents will be in a state of shock because they were not expecting it.

The sensitivity with which we approach the family and make the arrangements on their behalf is heightened because we won't be sure how they are going to handle it. There's a spectrum of reactions and, sometimes, the medication some of the mothers will be taking following the death of their baby can leave them either very numb or at the other end of that spectrum where they just cannot cope with it.

Not coping can show up in all sorts of ways: denial that it has happened, not accepting the circumstances, not accepting the death, not wanting to let the baby go, not wanting any support but, instead, going into themselves and internalising what has happened which can leave them very isolated. This can be a problem for us because it's then very difficult to get from them what they want. It's quite common that the mother will go into herself which leaves the father trying to make the decisions and hope they are the ones that will make her happy.

I think how someone grieves is very dependent on their upbringing and whether they had parents or other people around who helped them to develop their emotional boundaries or whether they were left to do that for themselves.

One of the biggest challenges for a parent who has lost a baby to stillbirth, or had a late miscarriage, is the challenge of letting go. They may want to come and see their baby in the Chapel of Rest, and we can support them with that, but at some point, they need to agree a time and date for the service and let their baby go.

We would never charge for a baby's funeral. Most people who are in that situation will not have prepared themselves financially or emotionally and so we feel we can provide a service and support to people who never expected to find themselves in this position. Most burial and cremation authorities don't charge either.

We have a real feeling of providing not just a figurative shoulder and an arm around the bereaved parents, but because it is such an intimate loss, there is a kind of tenderness to the feelings involved

Most parents will have a name for their baby, even if the pregnancy ended mid-term and we will use that name in the service. I think it's right to choose a name because it's a recognition that the parents and the baby have shared something, and that something was important to them, though, of course, not everyone wants to.

The provision for acknowledging the loss of a baby is far better than it used to be. There's more accountability and the days have gone where matron would have just spirited the dead baby away, never to be seen again.

The whole subject of death and dying has largely been, at least until recently, a taboo. It's something we're emotionally frightened of. But if there is a positive thing to have come out of social media, it is the opening up of people's perceptions of death and dying. We're better at dealing with end-of-life care for people with life-limiting illnesses. But the thing with baby loss is it's a short time frame – nine months if you get to term and often less than that – and frequently parents can't get an answer to why it has happened. So that leaves people, especially bereaved parents, flailing around.

The fact is people don't know what to say when a baby dies. They don't just avoid conversation, they will avoid contact with the bereaved parents. Sometimes though, you don't need to say anything. Sometimes you just need to sit there and listen.

And then, when the arrangements have been made, a funeral is an opportunity for people to mourn; it's an old word but there's still a need for that and for all of us to come together, feel connected to and respect for the people who have suffered a bereavement and, together, say goodbye to and lay to rest the child the parents had hoped for.

Whilst for many parents burial of their baby will happen quickly following their death, this information may help those parents choosing and planning a funeral at a slightly later time. For some this will not be a decision but a cultural necessity. Clive makes it clear that a ceremony, whether you decide to have your baby buried, cremated or create a ceremony of your own, is important both as a way to say goodbye to a hoped-for child and of respecting what the parents and their close family and friends have lost with the unexpected death of that baby, including those born pre-term.

If your baby died before birth and had not reached 24 weeks of pregnancy, you won't be able to register their birth officially. You can, however, request a special certificate from Sands or from the midwives which you will then need to show to the funeral director if you are arranging a service to say goodbye.

If your baby was stillborn at 24 weeks or later, or died after birth, you are legally required to have a burial or cremation for them, although not necessarily a funeral. Your baby's stillbirth, or birth and death, must be registered by the local registrar of births and deaths and the hospital staff will tell you how and where to register. The registrar will then give you the certificate that you will need for the burial or cremation.

Although there is no legal requirement to have a funeral, it is, as Clive says, an opportunity to come together with family and friends to mourn your loss. You can arrange the funeral yourself or you may prefer for the hospital to arrange it, in which case you will need to let them know that is your preference before you are discharged to go home. Some hospitals can arrange funerals only for those babies who died before birth and most funeral directors, like Clive, will offer a funeral free of charge for babies.

Like some of the parents who share their stories later in the book, it may be important for you to take your baby home with you before the funeral and again, as long as there has not been a post-mortem, this can be arranged with the medical team taking care of you.

Many hospitals give parents a form to take with them to confirm their right to take their baby's body out of the hospital. You may like to take your baby for a walk or to meet any other siblings, family or friends and you can ask for special permission and the paperwork to do this. If you do take your baby home, ask the hospital if you can borrow a cold cot (often called 'cuddle cots') which will help stop their body from deteriorating before the burial or cremation.

You can also arrange to take your baby out of hospital to visit a special place or arrange for family to visit and say hello and then goodbye to them. This is your baby; you are the parents so if there is something you think will help with your bonding and then the difficult task of letting go of your child, ask the experts, including the helpline advisors at Sands, to help you make that happen.

If you don't take your baby home, they will probably be kept in the maternity unit mortuary. Again, you can visit with them here but be aware, this will feel very different from spending time together in a private bereavement suite. Alternatively, your baby might be in a Chapel of Rest or a room by the mortuary that is for any adults, children and babies who have died, and so this too might feel more difficult for you. If the hospital is arranging the funeral, the staff will tell you when to bring your baby back or when to take them to the funeral director.

If you are arranging the funeral yourself and don't want a hearse to take your baby to the funeral, then tell the funeral director that. You can also collect your baby and take them to the ceremony yourself, but if you are using a taxi, make sure that they agree in advance to transport a coffin.

If your baby is at home, then of course, you can take them directly to the funeral.

For some bereaved parents, their baby's funeral will be the first funeral they have ever had to think about, and for some it will even be the first they have ever had to attend. Parents sometimes find that they want different things and so need time to reach joint decisions. Use this time to talk to family members and close friends about your choices.

If you have had twins or more babies from a multiple birth who have died, you may want them to share a coffin and a funeral. And if you have older children, you may want to include them in planning your baby's funeral (see page 141 for more on this). Likewise, if you have a surviving baby who is still in

43

hospital, you might like to wait until they recover so that you can take them to their sibling's funeral. If you need to arrange a funeral very quickly for religious or other reasons, please tell the hospital staff. They will advise you about urgent registration so that you can see if this is a possibility.

The most important thing when it comes to making decisions about the burial or cremation of your baby, and the funeral service or other ceremony you want in order to say goodbye and mourn that loss, is that the decisions you make feel right for you because there is no right or wrong thing to do and, as Clive says, a funeral service for a baby is a very personal and intimate thing.

There is a lot of information about funerals, burials and cremations on the Sands website, and you can also find out more about your rights at www.iccm-uk.com/iccm/downloads/, where there are downloadable documents about baby and infant funerals.

CHAPTER 3

Bereavement Support

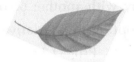

*'Group counselling is not right for you; you haven't
lost someone you loved.'*

Family GP to a grieving mother

This powerful and shocking quote thankfully does not reflect
common thought or practice and it is widely recognised that the
death of a baby is traumatic and that parents will indeed need
much support. The care that bereaved parents receive in hospital
following the death of their baby is crucial. These experiences
may be remembered by parents for the rest of their lives, and
bad experiences are likely to exacerbate feelings of pain and
grief for bereaved parents, potentially for many years to come.
Sadly, it remains the case that the standard of bereavement care
in the UK still varies hugely between regions making it something of a postcode lottery as to whether the hospital you attend

has a dedicated bereavement suite or even healthcare staff who have been trained specifically in the care of bereaved parents.

In a bid to tackle this inconsistency, the National Bereavement Care Pathway (NBCP) – a Sands-led initiative in collaboration with other charities, Royal Colleges and influencers and supported by the UK government's All-Party Parliamentary Group (APPG) on Baby Loss – was launched in October 2017. As of January 2020, there were 53 health trusts in England voluntarily signed up to the new pathway, with another 60 or so having expressed 'strong interest' in adopting the initiative.

Marc Harder, NBCP UK Project Lead at Sands, explains that: 'We want parents to be able to have time with their baby and we want parents to be offered those tangible things that help create those precious memories, which can be a cold cot which enables more time with the baby, or memory boxes, teddy bears, hand- and footprinting kits, equipment to take photos, etc.

'All of these elements are so important but their adoption, without the relevant sign-off within trusts from the various directors or heads of department, is still inconsistent. Of course, we'd love a bereavement suite in every hospital, but other departments and wards will have demands on resources and physical space. We'd also love every member of staff who comes into contact with bereaved parents to be well trained, but that incurs cost as well.'

Bereavement Suites

As the stories throughout this book will show, small details in how bereaved parents are cared for in hospital – and even where they are cared for – make a huge difference to the memories of shocked and grieving parents who must leave hospital without their baby and then process those memories.

In a best-case scenario, which we know is not always possible because of the competing demands for funding that healthcare trusts must juggle, a hospital will have a dedicated bereavement suite which affords grieving parents privacy – an intimate space to bond with and then say goodbye to their baby with protection from the sounds of a normal labour ward. Even if an entire suite is not feasible, the hospital should provide a private room where the parents can start the grieving process and, if the baby has died in utero, give birth with all the support they would get on a normal labour ward.

Sands has published meticulous guidelines for hospitals that are keen to get this balance of providing specialist bereavement care alongside maternity services to families whose baby has died. These are so detailed they include suggesting even the label on the door identifying what the room or suite is reserved for should be discreet so that other parents who may be passing will not be alerted to the true purpose of the room.

Another crucial detail – and one that is hard to read if you have been protected from the reality of a baby dying until now – is the need for a cooling facility (sometimes called cold cots) so that parents can spend time bonding with their dead baby without having to make an emotionally challenging and very public trip to the mortuary to do so.

Ideally, Sands would like every hospital to have at least one dedicated bereavement care room or suite where parents can be cared for following the death of their baby, and to use these facilities not just for babies born dead at full-term or within the definition of a stillbirth (24 weeks' gestation in the UK) but also for parents who suffer a late miscarriage or an ectopic pregnancy or the sudden end of a first-trimester pregnancy. In other words, all and every baby loss needs specialist care and sensitive handling all of which, it has been shown, plays a critical role in helping bereaved parents to grieve their loss in as healthy a way as possible once they return home empty-handed.

Just as importantly, these dedicated rooms or bereavement suites should only be used in cases where parents have experienced or are likely to soon experience the death of their baby. They should be made as private and comfortable for both the parents and visiting family as possible and, again if possible, avoid the need for anyone involved to have to interface with the outside world just to go to the toilet or find refreshment. In other words, they should create a safe and respectful private 'bubble' which confers dignity to all involved and allows a family to meet and say goodbye to a dead baby without feeling rushed or that their presence is an unwanted inconvenience to staff, or an unwelcome reminder to other parents that things can and sometimes do go wrong and not everyone comes home from hospital with their baby.

Empathic Medical Care

'While no level of care can remove the grief that many parents will feel, good care can make a devastating experience feel more manageable while poor-quality or insensitively delivered care can compound and exacerbate the pain.'

Sands UK

Time and again, when speaking with bereaved parents, one of the biggest things that stood out, however their particular story had unfolded, was how the care they received from the health professionals running up to the birth, during and after made such an enormous difference to their grieving process, not only at the time they walk away from the hospital without a baby in their arms, but for many years later.

Imagine losing your baby and being given a leaflet called 'Unexpected Outcomes' to walk out with, instead of a child. Imagine looking into the eyes of a young, inexperienced midwife and thinking, 'She's more terrified than me.' Imagine being in the delivery suite waiting for an induced labour that you don't want, and you're not prepared for, to start. Imagine waiting for a baby you know is already dead to be born into utter silence. And imagine thinking, as one bereaved mum puts it so poignantly, 'I just want someone to hold my hand and say yes, this is rubbish.'

Worse, imagine being in that delivery suite having been relegated to the role of 'bystander almost-dad' and hearing the surgeons discussing the relative merits of their smartphones as you wait for the delivery of your dead twin boys and the breaking heart coming your way and that of their mother. Ask writer, bereaved dad and 'Shoebox of Memories' blogger, Richard Boyd, about that particular scenario because it happened – that's what those doctors were talking about during one of the worst and most devastating times of the couple's life.

And Richard heard every word.

Connection. Compassion. Empathy.

Can it really be that hard?

'I do remember the bizarre need to accompany a nurse with our boys across the ward to find a set of scales. I have no idea why they didn't just bring the scales to us rather than make us slink through the maternity ward afraid that I might bump into a new mother and scare her with our tiny unmoving children.'

Richard Boyd, bereaved father

Sands, along with others, invests in bereavement training workshops for midwives and this part of the book is in no way intended to undermine or fail to acknowledge the fantastic work midwives do in supporting women who bring their babies home and those who don't. But it is important to acknowledge too that the death of a baby impacts on health professionals and that specialist training for when things do go wrong is critical.

Being with mothers who experience late miscarriage, stillbirth, the death of their baby after just a few days, Termination of Pregnancy for Fetal Anomaly (TOPFA) or an ectopic pregnancy is emotionally challenging for health professionals, but good bereavement care is critical to the family in coming to terms with their loss and their recovery.

Midwives and others involved in bereavement care when a baby dies have to respect the individuality and diversity of parents' grief and validate the parents' feelings. In an article entitled 'Supporting women, families and care providers after stillbirth' (written for the *Lancet* medical journal's recent series on stillbirths), the authors urge midwives and other health professionals who have been involved to show that they too recognise and value the baby by using the child's name, provide information in a parent-centred way and enable the creation of memories for the parents.

'Staff need to show sensitivity and empathy, validate the

emotion of parents, provide clear information, and be aware that the timing of information could be distressing. Supportive bereavement care can help families deal with their loss but can also help the healthcare professional address their own feelings of distress and sadness after a stillbirth.

'Bereavement care and support for health-care providers is important in all contexts and countries. When such support is missing due to scarce resources, the burden of loss is even greater for the women and their families, as well as for the midwives, doctors and nurses who attend them. Attention must be given to the care of both families and the health professionals who attend them to ensure that the burden of grief after a stillbirth does not affect the capacity to provide quality care to women and new-born babies.'

In other words, it is not just the bereaved parents who need bereavement care; those health professionals affected by the death of that baby need it too.

Erica Stewart, whose Baby Shane died 37 years ago (see page 88 for her story) and who spent 25 years working at Sands as a bereavement co-ordinator, makes the point that caring for bereaved parents may not be the right thing for some midwives, either due to their own experiences or circumstances on the day. When Erica started working at Sands, midwives were not always trained to cope with the death of a baby; now most hospitals have a bereavement midwife who is responsible for both the training of staff and providing support when a baby dies.

'In an ideal world, midwives would be asked, "Are you OK to cope with delivering a baby that has died?" It might be they have had a bereavement in their own family, or it could be they've had a row with their husband that morning and so they're not in the right place to cope. I think they should be given a choice where possible.

'Sometimes, of course, the baby dies unexpectedly, but I do think more respect should be given to how they feel about it and they should feel free to be able to say, "Actually, I can't cope." Healthcare professionals dealing with a bereaved family need permission to speak up and say, "I'm not the best person to be doing this."

'It doesn't matter how much training they have, if you trigger something in someone that's going to be negative or get in the way of caring then they shouldn't be asked to do it. They should have permission to speak up for themselves.'

'Bereavement training must be included in midwifery education. Students are often protected from caring for families who have had a stillbirth because of their inexperience. Thus, student midwives have little preparation for stillbirths and are often unable to adequately support women or one another when the time comes to provide care. Stories from mothers and fathers who have experienced stillbirth can be a useful way to facilitate learning in midwifery education by giving students insight into the perspectives of affected families.'

From the 2011 *Lancet* series on stillbirth, published online 2016

We know it can be difficult to know what to say when a baby dies and, unfortunately, even now, parents who have this terrible experience wince when they talk of being on a labour ward and hearing the sounds of other babies crying. One bereaved mum sums this up painfully when she writes of having this all too common experience: 'It was torturous.' Another, describing the same trauma, says: 'It is like having a knife stuck into an already broken heart.'

Bereaved parents are generous. Many, having worked through their own grief, work tirelessly with organisations like Sands to campaign and fundraise to try to ensure fewer families will have to go through the same shattering experience of coming home from hospital without a baby. They also volunteer to support other families now coming to terms with the same thing and many work with and train health professionals to help improve understanding of the experience of the death of a baby and what will feel important to the parents and the family in the hospital setting when that happens.

So, they are not complaining because they begrudge the fact other families are having a better outcome – a live baby – they are simply asking for some empathy, and an understanding that a painful situation is going to be made excruciatingly more painful unless compassionate and private provision is made for them to have their baby, see their baby, make memories of their baby and say goodbye for good to their baby; all of which needs to happen away from the normal sounds and sights of a labour ward.

If you feel you did not have the empathic medical care you would have liked, it may make you feel better to take action, rather than be isolated in the privacy of your home, and when you are ready, put pen to paper and write to the health trust explaining what happened and what you feel could have been handled better. This will help you feel your voice is important and can be heard and, even better, may result in more empathic practices being introduced at that hospital which will help the next family going through a similar experience.

If you are not sure how to word your complaint or even who

to send it to, just pick up the phone and speak to someone at Sands who can advise you and, if you haven't already found it, direct you to your local support group which you may like to think about joining for additional support.

The good news is that specialist healthcare for bereaved parents is improving overall thanks to the efforts of bereaved parents who have spoken out, Sands and, of course, those health-care professionals who want to know how to make things better for bereaved parents and who have attended specialist training. Between 2018 and 2019, Sands facilitated training workshops for healthcare professionals at 145 different locations across the UK resulting in some 2700 attendees – in fact, every single person who took part – reporting the training was not only helpful to them but one they would recommend to colleagues: 'Brilliant training, really helpful,' said one midwife. 'I now feel much more confident in caring for these families.'

In addition to these training sessions, many of the Sands Befriender volunteers will give up their time to go into hospitals to talk to health professionals about their experiences of losing a baby and discuss what helps bereaved parents and what doesn't (see page 240 for more on Befrienders).

All the blankets in the Sands Memory Boxes are hand-knitted by volunteers around the country. These blankets are a very special part of the box and bring much comfort to parents after the death of their baby www.sands.org.uk/get-involved/volunteer-sands/knit-sands

BEREAVEMENT MIDWIVES

Marie, whose baby, Stanley, died just days after his birth, credits the specially trained bereavement midwife she saw monthly for a year with saving her life, describing that midwife as 'my angel'. Here is her story:

STANLEY: BORN 13 AUGUST 2008, DIED 18 AUGUST 2008

My menstrual cycles were awful, often going months without a period. The doctors said if we were not pregnant after two or three years then they would intervene. We were not in a rush but decided to throw caution to the wind, knowing pregnancy, without fertility treatment, would be a miracle.

Eight months after our wedding I realised I was pregnant. We were elated. We were young but secure with good jobs and a mortgage on our own home.

I bled at 9, 11 and 14 weeks. And each time, at the hospital, we were told to prepare for a miscarriage, although each time the scan showed our baby was doing fine.

Things settled and I enjoyed the pregnancy and planning for our new life with a baby. At 22 weeks, I had a massive bleed at work. At hospital they said there was nothing they could do for our baby (as the pregnancy was not legally viable) but told me to rest. At 23 weeks and 6 days I had another massive bleed in the early hours of the morning. We rushed to the hospital and this time, as I was only a day away from viability (24 weeks), they agreed to try to help me and our baby.

We needed a bed for me and an incubator in case I delivered early and eventually they found a bed for us in the hospital in Plymouth, close to our South Devon home. I stayed there for a week and, at 25 weeks, although still bleeding, they said I could go home for rest. I still don't know why I said it but I asked if I could stay one more night and they agreed.

At around 6pm I felt my baby moving around a lot. I was scared, and so they checked on me throughout the night. At 6am they said, 'You're 3-cm dilated and in labour.' My husband and mum raced to me from 25 miles away. At 11.08am I counted 11 people in the delivery room as I delivered. I looked down to see a tiny bottom sticking out and realised he was folded over coming out bum first. Although tiny, he had long arms and legs and opened his eyes. He was whisked away. My placenta didn't come out, so they whisked me to theatre. I screamed at my husband to follow baby Stanley who was heading to NICU. I realised after that he watched the whole thing and thought he was about to possibly lose his wife and son who were both seriously unwell.

So, our firstborn son was born at 25 weeks and 1 day, weighing just 1lb 11.5oz on 13 August 2008. I came out of surgery and was wheeled to a six-bed ward at around 6pm. As they were moving all the machines about, I was handed a Polaroid of Stanley in an incubator and told he was in intensive care. The emotion and trauma of it all suddenly hit me, and I found myself sobbing hysterically quite loudly so was moved to a side room.

I was told the next 24 hours would be critical for Stanley but that he was stable. He did well and I was taken (in a wheelchair) to meet him. He was so tiny and there were so many machines on him I felt an overwhelming sense of wanting to protect my tiny baby. Later, a midwife handed me an A4 paper sheet showing diagrams of how to hand express milk. I was completely baffled – I'd had no baby classes or anything yet on how to deliver or feed or look after a baby. I was winging it. They came back and saw I'd not managed it and leant over and squeezed my breast a few times and went off with the colostrum. The next day they asked me to used Bertha – the large and loud breast pump – every four hours day and night.

My goodness the milk came in! In abundance!! I felt proud I could do this as a mother as I couldn't do anything else. At breakfast other mothers would wheel their babies in but mine was still in intensive care. I remember a mum showing off the eternity ring she'd been bought.

Things went downhill quickly. At three days old, Stanley suffered a bleed to his brain and was fitting. The consultant called me and my husband to a side room and said he would have cerebral palsy and possibly other issues, but he was still fighting. By day four, he'd suffered more bleeds to his brain and was having a difficult time. They said they'd continue to monitor and scan him, but we had to be prepared he could be severely disabled. I heard this horrendous wailing and realised it was coming from me. Never have I heard such a sound. Maybe I knew it was the beginning of the end . . .

On day five, I went to visit Stanley in the early hours having sat and pumped 3oz of milk. Nurses were all around him and there was lots of fuss. We were told he'd had a bad night and the consultant would chat with us. That morning, they said he was very, very unwell. His brain had swelled so much he needed an operation to relieve the pressure in his skull, but it was unlikely he'd survive the operation and would die in theatre. Or, they could start palliative care and we would need to give permission for his life support to be switched off. In that moment, without any discussion, my husband and I, at the same time, said, he's fought so hard we don't want him dying alone, we will switch off the machines.

We were told he could die anywhere between a couple of hours to a couple of days after coming off support. I was terrified it would be two days, thinking I can't watch him die for two days. After our parents said their goodbyes to Stanley, he came off the machines at 4pm. Finally, in a double bedroom, privately, we were a family, holding and cuddling our beautiful brave boy.

He opened his eyes for us and lay sweetly on our chests. We bathed him, dressed him and talked to him. They ordered pizza for us to eat! It was amazing to have our son to ourselves. I remember needing a wee but told my husband I'd go in the corner in a cup as I couldn't leave!! What if he died when I left!! I've never run so fast down a corridor to go to the loo!

At around 10pm, they checked on us and said it wouldn't be much longer as his breathing had tired. He lay on my chest, skin to skin, with my husband lying next to us holding his hand. I remember going to a place that was beautiful and white, cradling him in my arms. Peaceful and serene, I walked up a long path and saw my nan and lots of other people and animals. So calm. I handed him over and said, 'Look after him for me.' I turned and walked away.

At that point I heard the words, 'What did you say?' I woke to see my husband looking at me. He said, 'Marie, it's been a while but a few minutes ago he opened his eyes and just stared at me then closed them.' As soon as he said that, Stanley gave a large gasp. They say about that feeling of being stabbed in the heart and at that moment I got that. We held him, and his arms and legs now flopped either side of him and his colour drained.

For a long time, I never spoke about this 'dream'. I was a bit embarrassed. Did it happen? Was I asleep? But now it gives me comfort that I carried my boy over. One of the things I had said to the consultant when deciding on palliative care was, 'I carried him into this world, it's my job to carry him out.' It seems I did just that.

Six days we had him.

I've never held my husband so tight than that night we slept, after he died just past midnight.

That was the easy part. Leaving the hospital past all the happy well-wishers with balloons and flowers for other families, my legs stopped working. Driving home in silence. My husband sobbed for two weeks until the funeral. I went into planning mode. We had to register his birth and death to be allowed to bury him. The funeral; the absolute agony on my mother's face who couldn't make it better for her child, me. My tough father-in-law, who fixes things as the man of the family, wearing black sunglasses in the church and bent over double trying to keep it in.

I was fortunate to have the bereavement midwife who was with us at the end come and see me monthly for sessions for over a year after. She was my angel and I credit her for saving my life. She taught me what I was feeling was normal and how to deal with life. Those two hours every month were a lifeline. The first thing she'd said to me when we had met during palliative care was, 'Oh my God, you're the same age as my daughter.' I think that's why I felt so good talking to her.

Since the death of her firstborn son, who was named after husband Colum's grandfather, the couple have had two more sons, Erick and Frank. Marie says that bereavement counselling helped her come to terms with Stanley's death and grow around her grief.

Sands Support Groups

Sands volunteers now run over 100 support meetings every month across the UK and organise memorial events throughout the year around the country.

We've seen how important bereavement support is, both as part of the healing and a way to navigate to a new normal after a baby has died, and that this process starts at the moment you know your baby will or has died. We know empathic medical care will be important to you as you think about what has happened and we also know, at some point, you have had to leave the hospital and go home without your baby and often without any specialist support in place for when you get home and have to face your enormous loss.

For all of us, whether we have had good, empathic medical care at hospital or not, this is a very daunting time. Your life has suddenly changed and not in the way you had envisaged because the baby you were expecting to bring home is not with you. Family and friends will be devastated by your loss and, while they want to support you, they may feel very scared of doing or saying the wrong thing. You may have lost your partner into their own version of grief and you may now be feeling very alone.

If you have not done so already, you may, now you are home, feel ready to make a call to Sands to talk to someone who understands this whirlwind of confusing feelings you have been left with. You can talk through your support options which may include weekly counselling and/or joining your local Sands support group where you will be able to talk honestly about how hard this is and how horrible you feel.

As soon as you contact the Sands Bereavement Team you will be able to speak to someone who understands what you are facing and, from that point on, there will be someone who knows your name and your story and not only how hard the grieving process will be but some of the steps you can take to make it easier on yourself.

In the first few weeks you may just take one step at a time or accomplish one small task, and that is enough. Many aspects of life will just feel like hurdles to overcome and you may not find any joy or positivity in anything. This is very normal.

Sands staff and volunteer supporters recognise this may be all you can manage when you first come home without your baby, but they also know that all bereaved parents eventually grow around their grief to find a new normal which exists alongside the meaningful ways they find to create an enduring bond with the baby they never got to bring home. But they also know these changes can only happen in baby steps – at your pace and only when you are ready.

TWINS AND MULTIPLE LOSSES

If you have had twins or multiple babies, you may be facing a situation where all of your babies died, or one or more is still alive. And if the babies who are still alive are also unwell and in neonatal care, you will feel exhausted trying to focus on their needs, while also grieving for the baby or babies who have died. Sometimes twins or multiples who are unwell may be in different specialist centres in different parts of the country which makes visiting them, while also trying to manage the practical and emotional aspects of your grief, extremely difficult.

If you are trying to manage in one of these situations, please ask for help. It will be difficult not to feel torn in all directions and as if you are at the mercy of the full range of emotions – from elation over having a baby who has survived to devastation over the death of the baby or babies who died. You may feel you don't know where best to invest your emotional energy and having someone – other than your partner or other family member who is also grieving – to talk to about the tsunami of emotions threatening, at times, to overwhelm you will help you to carry the burden of such mixed feelings.

Bereavement Counselling

Sands has helped lead the Baby Loss Awareness Week campaign for free psychological support to be offered to all bereaved parents, but until that happens there are really just two routes to finding a bereavement counsellor who will help you to navigate and integrate your grief following the death of your baby.

You can ask your doctor for a referral, but you may find it difficult to tolerate any kind of delay between asking for and getting an appointment, or you may decide to take the private route and pay for your own counselling.

A good starting place to find a bereavement counsellor in your area is to contact the British Association for Counselling and Psychotherapy (BACP) which has some 60,000 active members. Make sure the counsellor you choose is a good 'fit' for you and not afraid of the powerful emotions the death of a baby can unleash. If you are in a relationship, it is also a good idea to check whether you can have joint sessions with both parents and solo sessions on your own, where you will be able to explore your feelings without the fear of upsetting or worrying your partner.

Good Social Support

'Friends with children had no clue how to react to our loss and seemed to avoid us, while women heavy with child swerved from our company unable or unwilling to face the risk of sharing our reality. We learned the meaning of the platitude "words fail me". Same reaction with friends and social network; people feel it so viscerally, like wincing when they see a car crash, their words fail them . . .'

Declan, bereaved dad

Reports on the social impact and the support (or lack of) that parents receive after loss is mixed with both cultural 'norms' and attitudes playing a key role in diminishing the perceived value of a stillborn baby in society. The presence of strong social support is undoubtedly a protective factor against negative long-term outcomes for parents, but so is individual resilience. Intimate relationships are important too – and, if lacking or poor-quality, will result, according to researchers, in higher levels of both anxiety and depression among bereaved parents and relationship breakdown.

One thing that has changed dramatically in the last decade in terms of the support of a wider social network is social media and, for the generation that has grown up with the habit of sharing every detail of their life (albeit edited), from holiday photos to broken relationships, on their preferred social media platforms, there is nothing unusual about taking straight to those platforms when their baby dies.

Within seconds, a young bereaved mum can find a WhatsApp or Facebook group and talk to other mums struggling to come to terms with the death of their baby. And this means a new kind of support is instantly available to bereaved parents who are comfortable taking that route. This is the kind of support that can help a newly bereaved parent feel heard and not alone in their grief which is important. It may be that, in addition to peer support, further counselling feels necessary and this may be at any point during your bereavement. Someone trained in baby loss counselling will provide a safe and boundaried space for you to explore your feelings and help you find your way to a new normal.

CHAPTER 4

Growing Around Grief

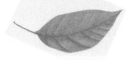

'There is a crack in everything. That's how the light gets in.'

Leonard Cohen

While there are clearly defined stages of grief, what makes the bereavement experience so difficult to manage is that recovery is not a linear journey. You don't, unfortunately, move in a straight line from the first of the five stages of grief to the last and then know you are 'better'. Instead, grief can wash over you in waves and you will find yourself oscillating between the various stages, often feeling 'hijacked' by the intensity of your grief and how much it still hurts, even when weeks and months and years have passed.

That said, it is helpful to understand what the accepted stages of grief are and to be able to recognise when you feel stuck in one of those stages and at the mercy of the emotions associated with that stage. It is also important to know that, although you may not feel you are making progress with each day that passes since your baby died, you will be; just not in a nice, neat, straight line.

The late Swiss-American psychiatrist, Elisabeth Kübler-Ross, identified five key stages of grief, namely:

1 denial

2 anger

3 bargaining

4 depression

5 acceptance

These stages – as all of us who have been bereaved following the death of a baby or any loved one know from experience – do not necessarily happen one after the other; you might find yourself at any stage at any time, you may go two stages backwards, skip one or perhaps experience a combination of any of the stages at the same time.

Another of the grief models that the bereavement counsellors and Befrienders at Sands talk about is Dr Lois Tonkin's model which challenges the idea that time heals all wounds and grief diminishes over time.* It doesn't. But what does happen is you grow emotionally and, as you move through your life, you keep growing so that your grief no longer dominates your life to the extent it did when your baby first died.

---

* Dr Tonkin is a counselling lecturer at the University of Canterbury, New Zealand and has been an educator on loss and grief issues for a quarter of a century. She is also the author of *Motherhood Missed*, a collection of stories of loss and living from women who are childless by circumstance not choice.

Dr Tonkin has been teaching this model for 20 years and when you first learn about it, it will reflect where you are in the grieving process. For newly bereaved parents, it is probably an idea to park for now. But if your relationship with grief is now an old, even a comfortable, one, you'll be shouting from the rooftops: 'Yes, that's exactly it. That's what happens.'

The best way to describe this model of grief is to imagine a Tonkin or Kilner jar. When your baby dies, at that moment grief begins its terrible onslaught, that's all there is in the jar: pain, sorrow, fury, yearning, bitterness, anguish and misery. But, as time passes, your life will start to expand which means you (the jar) get a little bigger. Now, when you imagine that jar which was stuffed full of terrible feelings, there's a little more space. Maybe the jar is only two thirds full. Maybe the next time you look you've expanded so much there's just a pitiful pile of grief stuck to the bottom of the jar. It's still there. It's still the exact same amount of grief you started with in the first jar, but because the jar is so much bigger it appears greatly reduced.

Sometimes this model of grief is called the 'fried egg model'. Instead of a jar, imagine a circle shaded entirely by a yellow crayon. This is the grief of the newly bereaved. With time, the circle (you) expands and gets bigger and bigger (just like the jars got bigger) but the yellow 'yolk' in the centre, which completely dominated the first circle, stays the same size. Eventually, there is so much more 'white' than 'yolk'.

This then is the idea of 'growing around grief'.

It is not a process you can hurry or abandon. It will require hard work, patience (with yourself) and trust in the process. There will be times – like anniversaries or further bereavements – when it feels as though the jar has filled up again or the yolk has expanded and, even if this is the case, your only job will be to keep growing, around that grief.

So, how do you grow? How do you get to a bigger jar or an enormous fried egg?

Life does not stop when your baby dies. You may have stopped and will even likely feel highly resistant to the idea of 'moving on' and away from the pain and sorrow because it will feel disloyal to your child to do that. But unless you stay locked up in the fortress with that unwelcome roomie, grief, your life *will* expand. You may meet new people, have new experiences, find fleeting moments of happiness that will become less fleeting over time, even when your baby is not with you. Maybe you will find the courage to fall pregnant again and have more children; maybe you already had children who need you to go on (see Chapters 12 and 7 for more on this).

As you grow around your grief, you may learn more about yourself; what matters to you and what you can do to acknowledge the baby who is not with you while still living a life. You may feel for a long time it's not much of a life. It's not life with a capital L, and certainly not the one you – and your partner if you have one – had imagined or hoped for when that pregnancy test turned positive. But for as long as you are breathing, even if, for months on end, you are simply going through the motions and faking any sense of being all right, you have a life.

And by the way, it is OK, more than OK, to not be all right, not in the slightest. Your baby is gone, and you cannot do anything to turn back time and change that outcome. You will be dealing with a tsunami of difficult feelings, including perhaps feelings of shame and guilt (see Chapter 5), and you will be desperate for answers to questions that may not have any. Why?

Why did this happen? Why did it happen to me? What should or could we have done differently?

One mother told me when we were speaking about the challenge of grief that if you think about it, the death of a baby shares more than a passing relationship to the death of someone following suicide. Stigma is a key feature of both, society does not really want to talk about either and with both experiences you think you could or should have known and done something to prevent these deaths.

The old you may cling, at first, to questions of blame, and rights and wrongs. The old you may spend the early days trying to block out such difficult feelings coming at you all at once. The new you is not here yet. Expanding and growing around your grief requires the gift of time passing. And, until time has passed, it can feel as if the intensity of the grief will never pass either because, even with sensitive and supportive care, the grief that follows a baby's death can remain for a long time.

It is normal to experience strong emotions of sadness and loss, but you may find that your grief lasts a lot longer than you expect. You may already know someone who has experienced the death of a baby or you may have had this experience previously, but comparing your grief to that of another parent, or to even to yourself during a different baby loss, may not be helpful as each bereavement is unique and everyone grieves differently.

You might, however, find it beneficial to talk about your experience, especially if you are still finding it hard to manage everyday life or to work after several months. You may want to make an appointment with your GP to explain how you are feeling. They may refer you for specialist mental health support

if they feel this is necessary and you could also explore counselling, though many parents find specialist peer support is
enough to help them feel more 'normal' in their particular type
of grief.

The old models of grief may have insisted that you move on
and leave the baby you loved but never got to bring home behind,
but the new models of grief are all about creating an enduring
bond which will allow you to still love and cherish your baby,
miss them and even feel sad that they died every day, but have
a happy and healthy life moving forwards. And the single most
effective way of doing that is to talk to others who have found
what works for them.

*'Grief is love's souvenir. It's our proof that we once loved. Grief
is the receipt we wave in the air that says to the world: Look!
Love was once mine. I love well. Here is my proof that I paid
the price.'*

Glennon Doyle, author of *Carry On, Warrior*

A LOST FUTURE

It is one thing to grieve and mourn the loss of someone you
knew, loved, spoke with, made memories with and miss having
in your life. It is another to have the same deep feelings of grief
about the loss of someone you never got to know and, in many
ways, when a baby dies, this is one of the hardest things to come
to terms with: the feeling of having been cheated of knowing
who that baby would have become.

What would their voice have sounded like? Who would they

have looked like? What would they have grown up to do for work? What would have made them laugh or cry or get cross? Who would they have loved? What tapestry would they have woven for their life? How would your relationship have been with them as you raised them for independence and adulthood?

What all bereaved parents know is that when a baby dies, so does their imagined future with that child. There may already be other children in the family (see Chapter 7) or children that follow for whom you will be able to answer all the questions above, but for the baby who does not come home with you after birth, the only possible future relationship is the one you forge through your grief and nurture in your imagination. No wonder then that intense yearning is a key feature of the complicated grief that can follow the death of a baby; you will be yearning for something – somebody – that you cannot have, touch, hug or know.

Time will pass, as time must and does and, with its passing, your questions will change. Would that child have gone on to have children of their own? You may find yourself becoming a grandparent to the children of the children you have raised but you will feel, all over again, that you have been cheated of becoming a grandparent to the children of the baby who died and never got the chance of life.

Complicated Grief

Getting stuck in any of the five stages of grief we described earlier is not uncommon, especially when a bereavement has been sudden, leaving you with no time to prepare for the sorrow that follows. Grief counsellors, talk therapists, clinicians, academic researchers and others engaged in the study and understanding of human psychology recognise this and have been debating for a decade or so whether there should be a new official diagnosis of a form of grief they call 'complicated grief', 'prolonged grief disorder' or 'traumatic grief'.

This new mental health condition was finally included in 2018 in the World Health Organization's (WHO) eleventh edition of the International Classification of Diseases (ICD-11) for the first time, where it is described as being 'characterised by core symptoms such as longing for and preoccupation with the deceased, along with emotional distress and significant functional impairment that persist beyond half a year after the loss of a significant other'.

In other words, if you are feeling stuck in any of the stages of grief, six months or more after the death of your baby, it might be that you are suffering from this more extreme form of bereavement.

It is now clear that, for some, grief, just like the healing of any wound, can be complicated and, when it is, the symptoms are both heightened and prolonged beyond the normal period someone would expect to be grieving.

This is important because, while 'normal' grief (I know it is tempting to ask who decides what is normal when it comes to grief and what does 'normal' even mean) does not require clinical intervention, complicated grief does. And we can (academically at least) answer the 'normal' question because studies show that for most bereaved people, the intensity of the grief they feel is fairly low by around six months after the death of a loved one. That does not mean the grief has vanished or been resolved, it simply means it has become better integrated into their lives and is no longer an obstacle to an ongoing life.

Studies show that about 10 per cent of bereaved people will struggle with complicated grief. These will almost always be people who have lost someone through disaster or violent death. Complicated grief, post-traumatic stress disorder (PTSD) and complex PTSD are higher amongst parents bereaved by the death of a child. These types of responses to bereavement require very different support and treatment, but they are not yet always recognised by those providing services as being needed following baby loss.

One of the statements I read in a huge review of the academic literature on complicated grief that was published almost 10 years ago, and long before the WHO included the new classification, stated: 'Many patients have been on treatment-seeking odysseys for years after the death of a loved one, receiving little help.'

The review cited a study of 243 individuals seeking treatment for complicated grief in Pittsburgh which reported that 85 per cent had previously sought treatment for grief. The majority had tried at least one form of medication and one form of counselling. Many had made multiple attempts to get help. Some reported being told they were 'coping as well as could be expected considering how difficult their loss had been'. Some were told that years and years after the life of the person they were mourning had ended. That's like being told, 'What did you expect?' or, worse, 'There's really nothing we can do for you.'

What the above citation tells us is that people suffering from complicated grief will already know there's something very wrong. They may have already experienced 'normal' grief and so will know something has gone badly awry. What they don't know is how to fix it and get back on track.

> The hallmark of post-traumatic stress disorder is fear. The hallmark of complicated grief is sadness and yearning.

If you suffer from complicated grief, and many bereaved parents will, then you will already know the unique symptoms. But for those trying to support grieving parents and struggling with their own sadness when a baby dies, they are worth spelling out and not least because they define a trajectory that may lead to feelings of (and actual) isolation and possibly wanting to die.

You may feel that you are not allowed to express this kind of despair this openly, especially when others are telling you that you have so much still to live for, but once you (and they) understand there is nothing aberrant about these feelings, which will likely be the most challenging you will ever experience and have to master, then empathy with a capital 'E' becomes a natural and supportive response (see the difference between empathy and sympathy on page 191).

Below are the key identified symptoms that will lead to a diagnosis of complicated grief – but only if your doctor or counsellor has heard of this new disorder:

- A strong yearning for your dead baby.
- Frequent thoughts or images of your dead baby.
- Troubling thoughts about the circumstances and consequences of your baby's death.

- Intense feelings of loneliness and emptiness.
- Sleep disturbance, major depression and anxiety.
- A feeling that life without your baby has no meaning.
- Feelings of guilt, shame and failure – what did you do wrong?
- Feeling isolated, isolating yourself.
- Persistent feelings of shock, disbelief, anger and bitterness about the death.
- Excessive avoidance – trying to stay away from anything that is a painful reminder that your baby died (like other pregnant women, babies and children).
- Excessive proximity – trying to feel closer to your dead baby which can sometimes express itself as wanting to die yourself, leading to serious suicidal thoughts.

When it comes to mental health conditions, clinicians are just as wary (rightly) of over-diagnosing as they are of under-diagnosing, but most people will feel relieved when their 'problem' is given a name and efficacious treatment identified. Complicated grief remains under-recognised and, as a result, under-treated which then causes continued distress and impairment. But once diagnosed, what are the treatment options?

We have seen that complicated grief is not the same as depression or PTSD, although symptoms may overlap, so treatment protocols need to be targeted to the individual. While studies remain largely inclusive about what type of treatment will work best, there is emerging evidence that talking therapies – especially targeted complicated grief psychotherapy – can be effective in helping a bereaved parent navigate the enormous challenges of complicated grief.

'A number of mothers recalled suicidal thoughts because of their desire to be with their baby.'

From the 2018 Lancet series on stillbirth

TALKING THERAPY

Fiona Gilmour is an arts psychotherapist (who shares her story of the death of her baby daughter, Aphra, on page 257) and has worked for more than 20 years in London with clients stricken by bereavement and grief, including and especially following the death of a baby.

She says talking therapy works because (if it's good therapy) it creates a safe and trusted space and will be a relationship where you are not going to have to censor yourself for fear of upsetting or infecting someone you love with your despair and grief.

'The work in psychotherapy, like the work through grief, is not linear,' Fiona explains. 'There is no timeframe with grief, as much as the rest of society wants there to be, and once you find that special space with a therapist where there is trust and the ground is solid, you have the freedom to be disorientated and lost and bewildered and, between you, over time, you will incubate something that is both related and not related.

'No good therapist is going to tell you to pull yourself together and get a grip; and therapy can be especially important for those who feel, with the passage of time, it's no longer appropriate to talk about their dead baby. The impact of these babies is huge and far-reaching right through the family and the generations. We know, too, the death of a baby can trigger the onset of latent psychological issues that may be the result of bereavement or trauma years before which will be adding a whole other layer into the grief.'

As we have seen, Sands has been campaigning for free psychological support for every family bereaved by baby loss. It is a worthwhile campaign and one that is gaining traction, but the truth is that your therapy will only be as good – and as effective – as the commitment you and your therapist make to it; the work you both put in and your patience in accepting it is not, as Fiona says, a linear process and you will inch your way forwards in baby steps to exploring and finding a way of integrating all your feelings about what has happened.

We know the emotional impact of baby loss is long-lasting and that the feelings of shock, numbness, anger, resentment, sadness, emptiness, guilt, self-blame, loss of self-esteem, and many other emotions, may be present for a long time. The key difference if you are trying to work out if you are suffering complicated grief is that you cannot stop the yearning for your dead baby and the grief has not lessened six months or more after your baby died. If this is you, please go and talk to your doctor or a specialist support organisation/qualified counsellor who can help you navigate through complicated grief.

ANGER

'The danger is by not finding a healthy outlet for it, anger leaks out in unexpected ways or finds its expression in hateful passive-aggression or, worse, depression where the rage turns inwards.'

Richard Boyd, bereaved father

Anger lies at the core of all bereavement but especially complicated grief where there is a danger it can take hold and get stuck. Bereaved parents, who with the passage of time have learned to channel this anger for the greater good, talk of its usefulness in fighting for change and especially change in practice and policy that will help reduce the number of preventable baby deaths; but most of us also admit there are times when our anger has no useful outlet and those are the times when we turn it in on ourselves, perpetuating the painful cycle of complicated grief.

Richard Boyd, a bereaved father whose twin sons died in utero and were born dead at 31 weeks following an induction of labour, has been blogging about that experience and exploring how grief has changed him and the way he now sees the world. One of the things that impressed me about Richard, both in his writing (see www.shoeboxfullofmemories.wordpress.com/) and when hearing him talk about being a bereaved parent, was the strong sense I had that he was not ashamed of his anger but had learned, for the most part, how to express it to challenge the status quo and push for change, as well as to support other bereaved parents. Below he writes eloquently, even furiously, about the role of his anger in complicated grief following the death of his baby sons.

NATHAN AND LINCOLN: BORN 19 OCTOBER 2011

Anger is at the core of my grief, it's something that is a constant companion. After the initial shock of hearing the words we all dread to hear it was there (there's no need to state them, we know them too well to have to say them again).

The sadness of knowing our sons, Nathan and Lincoln, had

78

died was undercut with a fierce anger at the injustice of it all. I was angry that not only did my wife have to suffer this terrible loss, she had to go through a grotesque parody of birth.

I was furious with the mothers-to-be smoking outside of the maternity ward as I scurried past them, voice hushed as I worked through the phone book to tell family and friends what had happened.

That flame intensified to an inferno when listening to surgeons chat blithely during the birth as I desperately tried to keep my wife awake, terrified that I would lose her too.

There was an anger at the way we were treated in the hospital, how we fell down the priority order of care and the poor experiences started to outweigh the good, threatening to overwhelm the acts of kindness that were there in the most unexpected places.

Anger is one of the expected reactions, it's there listed in the long-misunderstood stages of grief. For me, it's not a stage, more of a hub the other feelings surround. There's both comfort and danger in that.

The paradox is that even though anger is seen as an acceptable, even expected, part of grief, I'm often afraid of openly expressing it. It's tied up in a whole mess of history and, like a fire, anger can be self-sustaining, seeking the next available fuel, something to justify that feeling.

In the early years, I felt a cold comfort that what happened to us could not have been avoided, we were unlucky, the wrong end of every statistic. There was no plan, no way this could have been avoided. This was the rock I built my acceptance on. Immersing myself in the stories of others and hearing the echo of my experiences in their own turned that rock into quicksand and threatened to drown me.

Anger and depression are reflective of each other. Anger is a furious inferno capable of destroying all in its path and leaving behind only wreckage and dust. Depression is quicksand pulling everything under its deceptive flatness into an inescapable abyss.

Of the two, only the first can be harnessed for good. Depression produces nothing good. By its very nature it makes its home in a bleak wasteland where nothing grows, a merciless, pitiless non-existence. It doesn't produce art or action, its brutal numbness smothers creativity, buries hope.

Anger can be translated into action. Sometimes destruction is needed to wipe away the old structures that confine and allow something new, something better, to be built. It was anger that pushed me to do more in our boys' memory and take an active role in pushing for change and offering support which many have found it difficult to find. It's anger that makes me attend and speak at events to make sure my voice is heard so that more parents could be spared the agony of a preventable loss and receive the compassion they deserve.

It's anger over the fact that millions of babies are dying each year and effective prevention is strangled by a misguided belief that preventable deaths are inevitable. It's anger that cultural stigma works against the bereaved leaving them lonely, isolated and belittled.

It's always there, and much like my grief, it shifts and changes with time. Anger isn't a single emotion, it's often a tapestry and part of understanding; it is having the space to find the threads. Sometimes it's underpinned by fear, that what happened to us will happen again. It may be frustration that, even after solemn vows of lessons learned and never again, we still find ourselves hearing the same stories of avoidable loss, insensitivity and sometimes outright cruelty.

None of this has been easy; having the mental distance and tools to unpick anger rather than just react has taken a lot of work. It's taken a lot of time to no longer feel angry that my father refused to hold his grandchildren saying, 'They're not dolls.'

It's taken time to no longer react angrily to well-meant but awful attempts at consolation. Having spent so long telling the story of my sons, I forget how horrifying it is to hear for the first time.

To a certain extent this type of cathartic venting serves a useful purpose but there is a danger to that release of pressure. Blowing off steam is one thing but scalding someone with it may drive them away and leave them wary of offering condolences in the future, paranoid of saying the wrong thing. I have raged against moments like that and thoughtless words, but by trying to understand that what seemed natural for me may have been deeply unsettling for them, I'm starting to reach an uneasy acceptance.

Day by day, it gets a bit easier to manage these things as I practise different techniques and see the small changes slowly adding up to something more. I still get angry when I feel forced to justify why I feel sadness at the death of my babies. I'm not looking for a fix or magic words, there are none. Acknowledgment is enough to begin with. Let me save my anger for something more productive.

QUICK TEST ON WHETHER YOU NEED ADDITIONAL SUPPORT

1 How often do you find yourself yearning for your dead baby?

    a) Sometimes

    b) Every day

    c) All day, every day

2 On a scale of 0–10 with 0 representing no feelings of anger, how would you rate your feelings of anger over the fact your baby died?

    a) 0–3

    b) 3–7

    c) 7+

3 How often does your ongoing grief stop you from doing new things?

    a) Sometimes

    b) Most of the time

    c) All of the time

4 How often do you blame yourself for the fact your baby died?

    a) Never

    b) Sometimes

    c) I always blame myself

5 How much does your grief interfere with your ability to work?

    a) Never, work is a welcome distraction

    b) Sometimes, though less and less often

    c) I can't work; I'm too upset

6 How often do you think life without your baby has no meaning for you now?

    a) Never

    b) Sometimes

    c) All of the time

Your results

If you scored mostly (a) answers, then you may not need additional help and therapy as you may be starting to integrate your sorrow over the death of your baby and grow towards your new normal.

If you scored mostly (b) answers, then you may be already growing around your grief and learning to manage the waves that threaten to upend you. You are making progress and may not need additional support.

If you scored mostly (c) answers, then you may be suffering from complicated grief and in need of professional help to get you unstuck. Talk to your doctor, a Sands advisor and/or a therapist and ask for help in finding the ways to integrate your sadness into your everyday life without forgetting how much your baby means to you.

Getting Stuck in Grief

When my babies died, I did not turn to Sands or any other bereavement charity for support. Looking back now, I realise I was very afraid of getting 'stuck' in my grief, especially once I knew I had made the decision not to get pregnant again.

Jen Coates is the Director of Bereavement Support and Volunteering at the charity and only too aware that, for some bereaved parents, that feeling of getting stuck in the spirals of their complicated grief can be a risk.

The key, she says, to getting 'unstuck' is to work towards creating an enduring bond – *loving you from here* – which allows you to keep the memory of your baby alive and recognised while you work towards 'finding your new normal'.

'For me, the Tonkin growing around grief work is incredibly valuable, enabling parents to form enduring bonds with their babies which in turn helps them to remember within a new and healthy "normal".

'One important way of ensuring a healthy grieving process is in the immediate bereavement care at hospital, or at home if neonatally – although this last aspect is a challenge as there will be a need for police involvement with sudden infant death. Training and empowering health professionals and others to respond sensitively and hold the space for parents to make memories, take their baby home, introduce them at home or in hospital to those important to them all helps to set the scene for the subsequent bereavement journey.

'Another complication for bereaved parents is that almost all those memories that help in creating an enduring bond have to be made retrospectively so it can feel strange initially taking hand- and footprints and spending time with your baby but, in a way, it's overlaying memories on to an experience so it's not easy but it is so important for that enduring bond.'

Jen goes on to explore the difference between fixed and fluid types of remembrance. Recent initiatives by Sands have involved fewer 'fixed' notions of remembrance including, for example, the creation of an allotment. This brings a quality of 'ongoing life' to the experience of gathering, working with and talking to other bereaved parents and, just as importantly, an understanding of sustainability through the natural and cyclical seasons of growth, harvesting, senescence and regrowth that lie at the heart of any living enterprise.

For bereaved parents, it is a challenge finding that fluid – not fixed – pathway from grief, through growth to hope, but it can be done, as many of the stories that follow in the book will illustrate. It is important because this is the pathway that will take you out of the hinterland, through the thorny thicket of silence, across the bumpy terrains of complicated grief and on to the enduring bond you want to keep and cherish with your baby.

CHAPTER 5

Dealing with Other Emotions

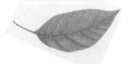

'There are so many difficult and challenging emotions – some may be familiar, but not all, which makes them even harder to cope with.'

Dr Clea Harmer, CEO of Sands

We know that the feelings which follow the death of a baby are strong and can be hard to talk about and share. Shock, numbness, anger, resentment, sadness, emptiness, guilt, self-blame, loss of self-esteem; any one of these feelings alone will present a challenge, but when a baby dies, many parents will experience what feels like a tsunami of negative feelings all jumbled together and all at the same time.

In one study of the psychological effects of stillbirth – the intangible costs – researchers reported that 70 per cent of mothers whose baby had died were still suffering clinically significant symptoms of depression, including anxiety, stress, panic attacks and suicidal thoughts, a year after their baby had died and half of these mothers were still suffering the same symptoms four years later.

In her story below, mum Erica, whose baby boy died at just eight weeks, describes those intense feelings of loss but also goes on to explore the less obvious feelings that can follow the death of a baby, feelings that can feel shameful to admit to but which are there nonetheless.

BABY SHANE: BORN 8 APRIL 1983

My name is Erica, and I am Baby Shane's mummy. Baby Shane died at eight weeks old on 29 May 1983. He had a complex heart defect and, following major heart surgery and much fighting for his life, he died.

It was a Sunday morning; I lay on the sofa drifting in and out of sleep. The phone rang, and it was a nurse telling me that she thought I should come in and give Baby Shane a cuddle. Little did I know it was to be the last cuddle I would ever give him.

We got to the hospital at about 9.30am; for three hours we took turns holding our baby . . . kissing him and cuddling him. He was still attached to the equipment that was helping him stay alive. We decided to go for a quick coffee break; we said that we would be back at 1pm – that was at 12.30pm. However, on the way out of the ICU, we met Baby

Shane's consultant; he explained there was nothing more they could do for him now.

We went for a coffee and returned at 1.15pm and, yes, you've guessed it, Baby Shane had died. He died at 1.10pm. In my mind, he had waited for 10 minutes, but we were too late. He died alone. For years I cursed that consultant, thinking if we had not met him in the corridor, we would have returned sooner, and would have been with our son when he died.

As I walked into the ICU; the doctor's face said it all! I remember I still followed the rules; I grabbed a gown and washed my hands with the special soap – I can still smell that Hibiscrub! Of course, on reflection, I needn't have done either of those things. My baby was dead; clean hands were not going to save him now. My son lay motionless on the ICU bed.

I picked him up and held him close to me, closer than I had ever been allowed to hold him before. Silent tears rolled down my face, and then Baby Shane's dad (also called Shane) held him in his arms, as I stood there stunned. I watched him as he wailed and rocked and wailed and rocked our son in his arms. I remember thinking at the time, 'I should be doing that!'

A voice asked me if I wanted to bath my dead baby. I declined thinking, 'Why does he need a bath, he's dead?' I watched as a nurse bathed my dead baby. Of course, now I wish I had bathed him, but at the time I felt rushed, confused and shocked!

They dressed Baby Shane in a white paper gown; his hands taped together holding a single lily. I noticed his tiny bruised hands, manhandled by doctors putting needles into him, in their bid to make him better, to save him. But his brow was now relaxed, no more frowning, no more fighting. He was peaceful now.

They put my baby in one of those see-through cots and put the three of us in a disused office. I remember standing there, staring at Baby Shane's chest, thinking I could see him breathing, hoping they had made a terrible mistake. Leaving hospital without my baby was one of the hardest things I have ever done in my life.

I remember that feeling of loss. I would look in drawers and be searching the house looking for 'something' I had lost. I didn't know what I was looking for, but God did I feel what I had lost. I felt incomplete, empty inside. The feeling to be maternal was overwhelming. I had been expressing milk for Baby Shane but now my T-shirt absorbed both the milk still leaking from my breasts, and my tears.

We organised the funeral ourselves; everyone wore white, as we had requested. This, we felt, reflected his pureness.

We scattered Baby Shane's ashes in the holy River Ganges in India, a place we had travelled to before.

Baby Shane lives on in my heart now. The waves of grief have got further apart, and I can speak about him without feeling that raw pain. I still shed a tear for him every now and again, but I wouldn't have it any other way.

My brave, brave boy, I love you, and miss you, always in my heart.

Love Mummy xxxxx

Erica goes on to explore the intense feelings of isolation the death of her baby triggered:

When you come out of hospital, you want the world to stop. If someone comes out of hospital after an accident and they have a big bandage around their head or they're on crutches, everyone can see and think, 'That looks painful, I wonder what happened?' But when you come out of hospital after your baby has died, nobody can see your grief – it's invisible. I remember wanting to shout out to the world 'MY BABY DIED'.

There's the lack of acknowledgement of the huge impact Baby Shane's death had, both in the wider world and amongst family and friends – that awful feeling of isolation where you're walking down the street and nobody knows that your baby has died – I wanted to say stop driving that car, stop talking to that person. I wanted the sun to stop shining – it should have been, and stayed, cold and miserable and raining.

Then there's the lack of acknowledgement from family and friends; they just stop talking about it. A lot of the mums I've spoken to tell me they feel like they've got a disease, people cross the road to avoid you, but you can imagine the whispers with them saying, 'There's that lady whose baby died.'

People's silence was very loud!

Guilt

If grief – the bully we met in Chapter 1 – has a lifelong bedfellow and playmate, it is his sly and constant companion, guilt. When your baby dies, you won't meet the one without, before too long, the other. Time and again, through all the stories parents have shared for this book, the second big 'G' word swiftly follows the grief word.

Mum Joanna Froud, who lost her twin boys, reveals how her feelings of guilt translated into a hatred of her own body which she blamed for their deaths. It doesn't matter that this guilt is irrational; it is powerful and very, very difficult to get past. (You can read Joanna's full story on page 123.)

Researchers have reported that many parents have persistent feelings of remorse or guilt over not being able to save their baby and, while there is no clinical evidence for their efficacy in this grieving population (bereaved parents suffering from complicated grief), in a US survey of bereaved mothers, some 40 per cent were prescribed psychiatric drugs to tackle their depression. The same survey noted the vast majority of bereaved parents questioned – over 80 per cent – turned to Internet forums for support, while a third joined offline support groups and half turned to healthcare professionals for support. One father, who had turned to the Internet told researchers: 'I find it easier to talk online, when I try and talk in person, I just cry.'

Stigma and Shame

'Perhaps the greatest obstacle to addressing stillbirths is stigma. The utter despair and hopelessness felt by families who suffer a stillbirth is often turned inwards to fuel feelings of shame and failure.'

From 'Stillbirths: ending an epidemic of grief', *The Lancet*, 2016

Stillbirth is a loss that is fraught with ambiguity. The death of a baby often gives rise to existential questions such as, 'Why did my baby die?' or, 'Am I being punished?', and may lead to a loss of faith in anything at all. The bereaved mother thinks, 'I am cursed,' and then believes that she is . . . and researchers acknowledge it can then take a lot to break this conviction. A parent's response to the death of their baby is often influenced by cultural factors and beliefs.

When a baby has died, parents who already have living children, or go on to have living children, will question how many children they have and should say they have; and for the first-time parent, there is also the doubt about whether they are a mother or a father at all.

For some bereaved mothers, the feelings of having failed to take a pregnancy to term and come home with a baby can lead to an ambiguous relationship with their own bodies. And even if a mother can resist this, there is the nagging suspicion many bereaved mothers admit to, that others may blame them in some way for the loss of the baby.

'For a long time, I couldn't look people in the eye because, when your baby dies, the feelings you have range from being broken-hearted and devastated to fury and anger, but you feel

93

a bit ashamed as well. You feel like your body hasn't done what it's supposed to do; and you've not done the only job you're supposed to do as a parent, which is to keep that baby safe. It took a really long time for me to be able to lift my head again.'

Janine Morris, bereaved mum

Bereavement psychotherapist, Fiona Gilmour, has spent over two decades working with bereaved parents and thinking about those more difficult feelings – including guilt and shame – that seem to plague bereaved parents following the death of their baby.

She told me of a time she was living in Ireland where she first came across a *cillín* burial site which was reserved primarily for stillborn and unbaptised infants who were not allowed in consecrated churchyards.

'It was extremely distressing; the energy was palpable and very sad, and it made me extremely angry too,' she recalls. 'I was thinking how shameful this must have felt – to have your baby die and then be excluded by the Church, and your community, from any blessing or support.

'I remember being overwhelmed for many years with feelings of self-blame when my baby daughter, Aphra, died. I can now see how my guilt and sense of failure tied into the cultural burden that a lot of women carry – that there is something wrong with you if you can't have a healthy and happy baby. It takes years to fully forgive yourself and make peace and deconstruct all the layers of internalised conditioning.

'And I'm not surprised that bereaved parents themselves are so reluctant to talk about these difficult feelings, even though there is much improved general encouragement to do so from bereavement midwives, counsellors, family members, etc. and all the charities now working with perinatal loss and the emotional quagmire that surrounds death. And yet we are not that far away from the time it was common practice to take stillborn babies away from their mothers and for the mother to never know what place their baby had been taken to. It's still very slow to deconstruct these patterns – it's like learning to speak a new language.'

Isolation

'People still find it hard to talk about death and dying gener-ally and the tragedy of a baby dying at what should be the most joyous moment is often too much for people to compre-hend. Many people do not understand that stillbirths and neonatal deaths happen as frequently as they do. People are frightened to say the wrong thing or upset parents/siblings, but the worst has already happened, and fumbled condolences mean so much when others avoid and add to the crippling isolation that can follow the death of a baby.'

Jen Coates, Director of Bereavement Support
and Volunteering, Sands

It is inevitable, following the death of a baby, especially a first-born before other children come into the family, that friendship circles may change with bereaved parents feeling they no longer fit with other families. At the start of the journey of complicated grief, it may be just too painful for bereaved parents to be around other 'happy families' celebrating a new pregnancy or the arrival of a new baby, and adopting avoidant behaviours to these triggers of even more painful feelings can leave a bereaved parent feeling even more isolated with their grief.

For many people, isolation, while understandable, is not good. It can be a short step from isolation – self-imposed or otherwise – to depression and a long hike back out from there. When a baby dies, your world view, your understanding of life and your self-esteem, even your sense of identity, all change too and it's not easy navigating so much change through uncharted territory. This is where, for some bereaved parents, connecting with others who have experienced all those same challenging feelings can prove a vital life support to help stop the spiral from isolation to depression. That said, what works for one person doesn't work for another. Parents may very well be at different stages of their grief; one ready to talk, the other still shut down.

For family members becoming aware of this alarming spiral, knowing what to do or say to halt it can be a challenge too, as can a growing and foreboding sense that they are now witnessing a loved one – a bereaved child, sibling or other relative – catapulted into the path of additional serious mental health disorders; additional to and frequently a big part of complicated grief.

What won't help is ignoring the spiral or pretending it's not happening. Bereaved parents often unwittingly become overnight experts in 'censorship', treading carefully with words and actions so as not to upset – sometimes it feels more like 'infect' – those who care about them with their intense grief and inability to cope or function as they did before their baby died.

One of the bereaved mums I spoke to for this book, whose social media awareness campaigns about baby loss mean her local community knows her first daughter was stillborn, told me in passing of another mum whose third baby had been stillborn. And who, as a result, had not been able to face doing the school run for two years. When she did resume, she fell pregnant with her fourth child and was astounded when, as her pregnancy started to show, nobody said one word about it. Not one word.

Clearly, the onus should not be on the bereaved to find a way to do or say the right thing. The onus is on those who love them to find something that might help. And acknowledging that a woman who has lost a baby but has found the courage to try again, just by saying the normal things you would say to anyone who is pregnant – 'Congratulations, when is the baby due?' – would be a good first step.

'This perceived lack of social understanding left these mothers alone and uncomforted. Added to this, the silence was aggravated by the failure of friends and family to acknowledge the loss and grief as real. They experienced people avoiding them, or treating them as though they had never been a mother.'

From the 2018 *Lancet* series on stillbirth

Grief is bad enough but a grief that the rest of society refuses to acknowledge as valid simply compounds the difficult task of recovery. It is distressing when both your motherhood and your baby are not acknowledged by others. One bereaved mother told researchers exploring the psychological cost of stillbirth that when she had told her sister she wasn't sure what to do about Mother's Day, her sister replied: 'Well, you're not a mother – you have to have your baby first.'

She *had* had her baby. Her baby had died.

Not surprisingly, bereaved mothers struggle with their own

sense of identity following the death of a baby because although they feel they *are* mothers, they are, if the baby was a firstborn, mothers without evidence of their motherhood; a status that is reinforced by the attitudes of others. One bereaved mother told researchers: 'If women haven't gone through a stillbirth, they don't want to hear about my birth, or what my daughter looked like or anything about my experience.'

Regret and Feeling You Made the Wrong Decisions

One of the themes that cropped up time and again when bereaved parents shared their stories for this book is that, while many of them felt 'something was wrong' towards the end of their pregnancy, they did not feel confident in identifying 'red flags' or, even if they did, they did not feel confident in knowing what, if anything, to do about them. Those mums who have talked about becoming aware their baby wasn't moving as much, if at all, didn't know whether they should go straight to hospital or adopt a wait-and-see approach. And for all those whose baby died, either before, during or soon after birth, and who were not given a clear-cut medical explanation for why, there is a very real risk they will default to blaming themselves.

When bereaved mum, Erica Stewart, first shared the story of the death of her baby, Shane, with me I was haunted by the poignancy of her regrets . . . missing the moment of Shane's death by just five minutes because a doctor stopped her in the corridor to say there was no hope; not understanding how the ritual of bathing him may have been an opportunity to create a lifelong memory of lovingly parenting him; opening the drawers and cupboards in her home after leaving hospital without her baby, desperately looking for 'something I had lost'.

Erica echoes the sentiments of so many bereaved parents who, reeling from the shock and distress of their baby's death, are in no position to make 'good' decisions. They simply cannot think straight. She, and the other parents who told me of living with the lifelong pain of the same kind of regrets, did not make 'bad' decisions. They simply found themselves catapulted into uncharted terrain (the hinterland) with so little time to spend with their dead child and no idea, without guidance or help, of how best to make those all-important decisions and memories that would mean so much later on.

We're beginning to see, as we explore not only the feelings the death of a baby will trigger but the bereavement support available when this happens to you or someone you care about, that asking for help and being encouraged to talk about what has happened is the single most important part of navigating this challenging mix of jumbled emotions.

Talking to a friend or family member is a way of embedding the baby and your experience in the family and the narratives of your wider social network, but talking to another bereaved parent, such as a Sands Befriender who has experienced – and survived – all these difficult feelings, will be more liberating because you don't have to worry about scaring or upsetting them.

You may decide to talk to a specialist bereavement counsellor or to join a Sands support group and talk to other parents, or you may just test the waters by joining an online forum and looking for answers and validation of your loss there. You may put together a combination of all these channels of support and dip in and out, depending on how you feel each day. But talking and being listened to is the proven way through this grief. There are no shortcuts but there are people who can hold your hand as you do this difficult work. You simply need to reach out to them.

CHAPTER 6

It's My Baby Too . . .

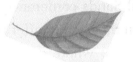

'Remember me, I'm here as well.'

A bereaved father's plea

We talk a lot about the impact of a baby dying on the mum but sometimes forget the non-birthing partner who will have been just as traumatised by the sudden end of a pregnancy and death of a baby, if not, in some ways, more so. For lots of partners, being relegated to the role of bystander when things start to go wrong means that the short- and longer-term impact of what they have witnessed isn't addressed.

A lot of dads, and other partners, talk about how scared they were that their wife or partner could die and many, especially if they have had no prior experience of birth or the labour ward, are left reeling from the shock of the blood loss, the panic, the drama and the silence that every bereaved parent talks of when their baby is born dead or dies during labour.

These experiences for dads and other life partners add up to a perfect storm of post-traumatic stress disorder (PTSD), which can often remain hidden because dads and life partners shoulder the burden of interfacing with the outside world, think it is their job to (and they want to) protect the mum and so they may struggle to find any place in this complicated landscape to deposit and explore their own trauma and feelings surrounding the death of their child.

At the 2019 annual Sands conference, entitled 'Finding Your Way', the focus was on the need to offer more support to fathers and included a workshop where dads were invited to suggest how the support they do get (oftentimes, none) could be improved. I sat in on that workshop and was shocked by the results of a Sands survey which explored the impact of a baby's death on men and women; and how men really felt.

Of those who had responded, 30 per cent of men said they had been offered no support at all and of those who had been offered some kind of support, only 13 per cent had been offered solo support.

'Everything was directed towards either my wife or together as a couple. I didn't want to ask for solo help on my own at the time as I know my wife would have just worried more at an already extremely tough time. From my experience it would have definitely helped if we could have had an "obligatory" solo conversation so I could have expressed my thoughts and feelings while not sat next to my wife. Instead, I just brushed them under the carpet and hid them, which hasn't helped me at all in the longer term.'

Bereaved father

More than half the dads who took part in the survey (54 per cent) saw their role as telling adult members of the family what had happened (bridging to the outside world) and almost half (49 per cent) believed their main role was to protect their partner; a huge difference from the 4 per cent of women who felt that was their job too.

Twice as many dads said they felt they had to 'put on a strong front' compared to mums who said the same, and a staggering 90 per cent of the dads taking part in the survey asserted that men and women grieve differently, with over 60 per cent stating it is more socially acceptable for women to talk about baby loss than it is for men.

When asked about feelings the bereaved couple were both having but not sharing – including anger, guilt, isolation and depression – again, a higher percentage of men than women admitted to keeping these difficult feelings to themselves. Alarmingly, the percentage of both parents unable to admit feeling suicidal either to their partner or anyone else was much closer, with 62 per cent of men keeping those feelings bottled up, compared with 59 per cent of women.

'I felt a duty to both protect my partner and yet to talk about what happened so as to reduce stigma. I felt shame, however, at being a victim of tragedy. I knew I had to be the stronger one at this stage of our relationship as my partner – the mother – needed me most. In some ways, this helped me. In others, not so much.'

Bereaved father

Another respondent, this time a bereaved grandmother talking about a bereaved grandfather, said this, which speaks volumes to the fact that the passage of time and another generation has done nothing to help men open up about their grief: 'The men don't know what to do with their grief. I found my husband sobbing on his own. He couldn't always reach out to me because he knew how it affected me. He felt his role was to protect and he couldn't protect our daughter, her husband and their child.'

What most of the fathers who spoke at the workshop I attended all said was that, in their experience, very few men – perhaps unlike the mums – would walk into a support group, sit in a circle and open up about their feelings, never mind admit to struggling with those feelings, when their baby has died.

'Men won't actively seek support for themselves and the very thought of a group therapy session, their perception of that and sitting in a circle talking about their feelings, simply terrifies them,' one dad told the Supporting Men workshop group, which was doing precisely that, sitting in a circle waiting for the dads to speak.

#stilladad

The fact is, while all the care may be geared up towards the mother, you both become parents in your mind from the very first positive pregnancy test. You start to imagine what life is going to be like with a new addition; the transition from being a couple to a family or the expansion of an existing family with the arrival of a new sibling. You create a space, in your heart and your mind, for this new arrival and begin the adjustment to the idea of a new person coming into your lives.

#stilladad is one of Sands' social media campaigns which aims to raise awareness that a dead baby will have had two parents and that means there are two people grieving, often from a gaping and huge emotional distance from each other; both struggling to make sense of the shock, the trauma, the disappointment, the difficult feelings that have been unleashed (guilt, anger, blame, shame, isolation and suicidal thoughts) and, ultimately, the loss of a shared dream.

And one thing all the men at the Sands conference workshop exploring the impact on dads agreed with was that the death of a baby puts an enormous strain on a relationship, however strong it was before the bereavement.

This is supported by research which reports that, where grieving is 'incongruent', marital disharmony can occur with both the physical and emotional relationship adversely affected. Research also shows that the risk of couple separation following a stillbirth is increased, which is not the case when a couple experiences the trauma of a pregnancy loss due to miscarriage. That said, many parents who have taken part in academic research actually report becoming closer through their shared bereavement, rather than growing apart. Bereaved father Matt's story below describes how the loss of their twin boys impacted his relationship with his wife, Joanna. At first, the couple – grieving in their own ways – felt like strangers to each other, but having worked through their grief, they found a way back to the marriage, went on to have two little girls and now have a marriage stronger than either of them could ever have imagined.

OLIVER AND JOSEPH: BORN 27 APRIL 2009

After an extremely difficult and complicated pregnancy, our gorgeous twin boys were born via C-section. Oliver weighed 1400 grams and Joseph a mere 635! They were rushed to intensive care. Six days later, we lost Joseph to NEC (necrotizing enterocolitis). At this point, Oliver was doing really well but two weeks later he also contracted NEC and we lost our second boy to the same disease.

We still cannot describe the desperate feeling of loss we both have in our hearts. From that point on, my wife and I really struggled with our extremely incompatible grief journeys. All my wife wanted to do was cry and talk, but I wasn't ready to talk. All I wanted to do was get back to work and keep busy.

The biggest thing that we have since learned from our experience is that grief is an extremely unique and personal thing. Understanding this at the time was impossible though. Neither of us could see it. Looking back on things now, it was as if we had hit a fork in the road on our journey. I wanted to take the left fork and my wife wanted to take the right.

Sometimes I felt as if I was being pulled down her road. She would spend days on end crying at home and looking at photos. All she really wanted me to do was comfort her and talk about the boys but, for some reason, I was unable to do either of these things.

I was grieving too but at the time she couldn't see that. It was as if she thought that I didn't care, and I just wanted to get back to normal. It wasn't that at all. I was constantly thinking about our boys. I just could not express it emotionally like she could. All I wanted was to keep moving. I was scared of what might happen if I stopped.

My first day back in the office was extremely difficult. I remember arriving in the car park and sitting in my car for a good 15 minutes before I gained enough courage to enter the building. Walking through those doors that day was daunting. I wanted people to acknowledge our loss but at the same time I remember trying to avoid as many people as I could.

I think I was scared what people would say and how I would react. I went straight to my office and tried to make myself look busy, but I just could not concentrate; my mind kept wandering, thinking about our boys, how my wife was coping for the first day on her own, and worrying about our failing relationship.

I wanted to go and get a coffee, but I wasn't ready to be around people chatting about their wonderful weekends. Even worse would have been a silence as I entered the kitchen. I just couldn't face it.

A few colleagues came over to my desk and expressed their condolences and welcomed me back to work. What shocked me the most was the ones I had expected to say something quite often didn't, and the ones I wouldn't have expected in a million years to mention it, seemed to make a special effort.

I now know how important it is to understand that we all grieve in extremely different ways, what may be helpful for one person is not always right for another, but it is only when you try all options available that you can find out what works best for you as an individual.

Eventually, our paths finally re-joined. We learned to deal with our loss as a couple and managed to move forward with our lives. Nine years on, we are a much happier and stronger couple and have since had two beautiful girls, Ellena, who is now seven, and Georgina, four.

Our beautiful boys will never be forgotten, and we talk about them every day. They are still a major part of our family and always will be . . .

The stress on couples when a baby dies can be huge. It can be difficult to give support and understanding to another person when you are so sad and in need of support yourself, and because grief is so individual, especially in the way that it comes and goes, it is likely that you and your partner won't feel the same things at the same time or want to express the feelings you do have in exactly the same way.

As Matt told us, Joanna wanted to talk about the boys all the time, whereas he wanted to crawl away and lick his wounds. The gap between a couple grieving can be so wide it is inevitable it will put a strain on the relationship. If you can, try to put your grief 'on hold' for short periods of time to concentrate on your partner and what they need from you. This is not easy and will take practice, but it will help keep the bond between you both going. And, of course, Sands can help support both parents through their grief when they are ready to reach out for that support.

Sands United

'When a baby dies, the feelings of loneliness and isolation can be overwhelming and having other bereaved parents to talk to is vital, but we know that dads can sometimes be overlooked or struggle to find support networks.'

Jen Coates, Director of Bereavement Support and Volunteering, Sands

Rob Allen is the founder of the first ever Sands United football team, which brings bereaved fathers together to keep the memory of their baby alive. They wear Sands United shirts with their dead baby's name in an embroidered heart and use their football camaraderie to open up a doorway to start to speak about and tackle those painful issues bereaved fathers face – including, and especially, finding it difficult to talk about their feelings in public.

The Sands United concept happened almost by accident, says Rob, who had no idea back in May 2018 when the first match was played that his daughter's still unexplained death, just four days before her due date, would lead to such a legacy not just for him and his wife, Charlotte, but for so many other bereaved dads.

NIAMH: BORN 9 OCTOBER 2017

In October 2017, we lost Niamh and had that experience of seeing a completely different side to the world. You live in blissful ignorance up until the point where you're exposed to something like that. The whole experience rocked and reshaped my outlook on my social life, so for a long time I didn't socialise. I didn't go out. I focused on the people who were most affected and most important to me which were the people inside my own house.

I stopped playing football for a while and then I got a call from my manager, Alan, who rang me in the January and said I've had this idea – me and the guys want to do something for you and the family.

Charlotte and I had been to a couple of Sands meetings at that point and so when Alan floated his idea about doing a charity football match to raise some money for Sands and do something for me and the family, I knew it was kind of their way of giving something back.

That's the difficulty for a lot of people – they don't know how to reach out; they don't know what to say or how to say it. And what they don't realise is that, actually, saying anything is better than saying nothing. So, this idea of a charity football match was Alan's way of reaching out and getting in contact with me. He probably had the same thoughts as everyone else: What do I say? How do I say it?

There are all these different thoughts and feelings, but there's no guidebook telling you what's right or wrong . . . so a lot of parents just get left to their own devices and sometimes that can result in a shutdown because other people just don't know how to approach it.

Anyway, Alan reached out to me and floated this idea and, although I still wasn't in the right kind of space to help out with it, I could see it would be a great opportunity to give back to Sands. A couple of weeks later, Alan called to say he'd only gone and booked the biggest football stadium in Northampton; the home of The Cobblers!

I liked his ambition and asked him who we were playing. At which point he told me he hadn't thought about that! By this time I'd been to quite a few Sands support group meetings and seen a few guys knocking about, although, to be honest, not many, but I'd seen lots of the women so I thought, well, behind each of these women is a guy who's just like me, so I told Alan I'd put a team of these dads together and play with them.

Rob was true to his word and put together a team of 17 dads; 15 of whom had lost their baby (the other two players were close friends with dads whose babies had died) and the first Sands United team stepped out on to the football pitch in May 2018 and raised £6000 for Sands. After just eight weeks of being formed as a team and with only a few training sessions (and with a team that included some players who had never really played football before but wanted to honour their child's memory), Sands United put in a very respectable performance having gone back into the match 1:0 up at half-time but eventually losing just 3:1 to the Eastern Eagles.

The idea of football as a way for bereaved dads to connect really captured the collective imagination and showed that many bereaved fathers would use the camaraderie of a shared sports activity to open a doorway to discussing deeper and more difficult feelings about the death of their baby which, for many, was also accompanied by the trauma of witnessing everything that happened in hospital and, at times, fearing the death of their partner through the labour.

Rob admits he had no idea Sands United would become so embedded in the charity and its fundraising efforts, or that other Sands United teams would spring up all over the country. He thought the lads might just keep in touch with the odd curry night or crazy golf outing, as well as through the dedicated WhatsApp group which he hoped would keep the bereaved dads, many of whom had not spoken to anyone before about their grief, opening up and talking to each other.

At the time of that first fundraising match, Rob says there was 'a void' for grieving dads in terms of any outlet to talk about their grief and accept their feelings:

'Mention a support group to most men and you'll get the vision of a turtle tucking its head back into a shell,' he says. 'Most men will just cringe and retract at the mention of the word "group".

'Nobody preps you for this experience, nobody knows what you can do to make the experience easier, so you just have to be brave enough to put yourself out there and experience what works for you and what doesn't,' he says. 'Being in a new situation means you have to try new things. You get out what you put in.'

Finding somewhere to talk about your feelings is a crucial part of navigating your grief as a parent, adds Rob, who uses a clever analogy of a bathtub filling with water to illustrate just how important 'owning your feelings' is: 'You have to let some of the water (your feelings) out from time to time or you'll flood and ruin your house.'

'What you have to do when your baby dies is learn your new normal,' he says, echoing what all the bereaved parents who contributed to this book have said. 'And that's the hardest thing of all. Your life will never be the same as it was before you lost your child but, on the flip side of that, and I say this because I am quite a positive person, that doesn't mean that experience has to define you or stop you finding the good quality of life that you can get back to.

'Niamh's death changed me, but the way it changed me was it made me determined to really live my life and honour her memory by doing that. I look at life completely differently now. I feel that I owe it to myself and to her to live it to my fullest. There may have been times before Niamh died when I may have held back or not got involved in things but, now, I feel I owe it to her to take every opportunity.

'I have to live life twice as hard; I have to do it once for myself and once for her. You never know what's around the corner so all I know is you just have to grab the throttle, grab life with both hands and go for it . . . and that's Niamh's real legacy to me.'

Rob's story teaches us two important things that challenge all bereaved parents who find themselves facing a new normal which was not something they had any say over. The first is that finding a new normal will demand that you step out of the comfort zone of your grief and try new things. Rob tried a support group and found that worked for him. He tried a fundraising football match and found that worked for everyone involved, including those players who were not bereaved and were struggling to find words to show they cared.

The second is that, in some way, every single baby that dies before, during or after birth leaves a legacy in the family. By living his life to the full, Rob wants to be twice the person he was before Niamh died and, for him, making that enduring commitment to his daughter's memory is a key part of sustaining his enduring love for and bond with her.

You don't have to join a support group, take up football, take part in a charity bungee jump or do anything that other people do to try something new and create a new normal, but you will need to be brave and find the courage to step out of your house, leave your grief behind for a while, and engage with the world in a way that will bring you new experiences and allow you to start that all-important process of growing around your grief.

Allen Family update: Fourteen months after their baby daughter, Niamh, died, Rob and Charlotte welcomed new daughter, Iris, after a long anxiety-filled pregnancy during which Charlotte told Rob she wished she could just be put to sleep and only woken up again to give birth.

'Every time my phone rang during that pregnancy and it was Charlotte, my initial reaction was panic! You're just waiting for that phone call that says something's gone wrong . . .' says Rob. 'You sit there quietly sweating through every scan because you don't want anyone else to know you're losing it . . . it's just horrible.'

(See Chapter 12 for more on just how anxious a subsequent pregnancy will be for bereaved parents, including dads.)

We've Never Really
Talked About This . . .

Rob and Charlotte have negotiated the challenge the grief and trauma of losing a baby dumps on bereaved parents and have gone on to expand their family with the birth of their second daughter, Iris, but not every couple manages to navigate that challenge and stay together.

For some of us, the loss, especially when there have been multiple losses, can create a chasm too big for any relationship to bridge and, in this section, we will explore the impact of baby death on relationships, sharing the story of one relationship that did not survive the trauma and one that did.

My ex-husband, Declan, and I went through the abrupt and traumatic ending of three mid-term pregnancies over a five-year period in my thirties and, while we eventually parted and divorced, we have found our way to a meaningful and supportive friendship over the years since then.

As I started this chapter exploring the impact of a baby dying on fathers, I realised I had never really spoken to Declan about how he had fared, either at the time those babies died or since. He already had a child from his first marriage so I had assumed he was, or would be, less devastated than me.

I noticed that whenever we did speak, he was showing more than a polite and passing interest in this book and I wondered if perhaps he wanted to write his story. When I asked him, he said yes, but then promptly disappeared, which I knew meant he was struggling to know where to start.

A blank page and a very emotional topic can be daunting, so I asked if it would help if I sent him some questions which then paved the way for us to have our first conversation in 30 years about the losses we had shared but not shared.

You could, if you are still together and even if you're not, put together your own list of questions for each other or even ask your partner, as I did, to tell your shared story in their own words (see the box below for some ideas). This can be a very useful exercise for you both, not when your baby has just died but when time has passed, life has moved on and when you perhaps don't talk as much as you once did about what happened and what you both lived through.

You will be amazed by what they write. I was when I read what Declan had written and by the fact that, all these years later, he sent it back with a poignant line which simply said: 'Susie, I found this very painful.'

SUSAN'S NOTES TO DECLAN

It's generally accepted all the focus is on the mum when the baby dies and that men and women grieve differently. I don't think the latter is true; I think the grief is the same but men find it harder to express because of pressures to be supportive, be a rock and, in particular, deal with/bridge back to the outside world.

Feelings common to both parents (and often expressed by neither) are of guilt, anger, shame and isolation so you could explore those if they are feelings you had. Also, impotence, in that you could not do anything to stop what happened or make it better afterwards.

You may have something to say about other people's reactions, e.g. 'It was the last thing our son needed,' (your ex-wife's response) or, 'Well, if there was something wrong with the baby . . .' (which people definitely said to me) or just their failure to find any words and acknowledge any loss.

You may have something to say about the toll it took on our relationship – because there's no question in my mind it finished me, or some other version of me.

- How often do you think about those babies who never were?
- Do you remember their names?
- Do you ever tell anyone about them? Does anyone close to you ever ask?
- Is time a healer?
- What happened to your own grief?
- Did anyone, throughout those experiences, ever ask, 'How are *you* doing?'

I know, for my part, I thought because you already had a child it was not the same devastation. Also, we did not share the disappointment of being childless. So, in some ways, that made me feel less guilty about my failure(s) but in others, it left me more estranged from you.

- Do you think of yourself as a 'bereaved parent', or do you think you don't qualify because the babies' deaths were not registered as stillbirths . . . or anything at all?

- Who did you blame or want to blame?
- Do you think the marriage would have lasted if we had not had those losses?
- Why do you think we have never really, in almost 30 years, spoken about it?

DECLAN'S STORY

My wife had three mid-term births, but our babies did not survive the trauma of birth or were too premature to live. The first was our baby, Boxer (nicknamed from his reactions during our first introduction by ultrasound). We were pleased to learn that we could conceive a child in the shake of a lamb's tail and stepped out on the path to parenthood.

The first storm clouds burst one afternoon when my wife returned early from work. She was ashen and worried, saying she felt something was not right. Within a short time of her return home, her waters broke. We were halfway through the pregnancy. I took hope from the absence of blood in the fluid. Our good friend, who was a GP, visited, examined and tried to soften the diagnosis, but his calm and quiet call to the emergency services to arrange for her admission into hospital betrayed his understanding that we were in the middle of a domestic tragedy.

Minutes grew into hours while we waited in the emergency obstetrics unit for confirmation that all would be well and modern medicine would work a routine miracle and restore the status quo – we were let down gently with the worst news imaginable as it was explained that there was insufficient amniotic fluid left for our baby to grow to term, the inevitability of infection, fatality and danger. We were told we would have to lose this baby in order to have a chance of having another that could reach full-term and viability.

We accepted the advice to kick-start labour and some-time, somewhere, during the next hours our baby Boxer stopped living.

After a very brief respite from the tempest of the real world, we emerged into that maelstrom and quickly realised that faux sympathy was readily available, while true empathy was in limited supply.

We shared our empty birthing and had a small capsule of time when we grieved together and poignantly attended a cremation for Boxer with one other mourner (my wife's best friend) and then took our baby's ashes home. We had been given some assurances by the doctors that this was an 'aber-rant' event likely due to an infection which could be and was now treated so, once we had drawn breath, we had no reason to doubt the certainty of a live birth following a further pregnancy.

My wife was trepidatious while I was eager to start our journey as soon as it was greenlit. Looking back, this mistiming of objectives opened up a crack within our rela-tionship that in time became a fissure. Perhaps unintentionally, our social network began to disintegrate.

The vacuum that our loss caused in our lives could not be filled by work or play and, in an effort to control our future by changing our scenery, we moved from the city to the home counties countryside and tried out new roles for size. This change allowed my wife to overcome her misgivings about pregnancy sufficiently to think about having a child again. In short order she was pregnant again and we embarked on this new journey as seasoned but optimistic travellers. This optimism was again misplaced because, at around the same time in this pregnancy, there was a serious bleed . . .

Our doctors explained that they could find no reason for this second mid-term loss, seeming to suggest it was 'just one of those things . . .' We were so disheartened and damaged by this second lightning strike that we found two different places within our relationship to lick our wounds and grieve for another baby.

At this point, it seems that the only other humans who can understand the pain are those experiencing childlessness as well. I did not share this, and our fissures deepened.

Attempts over the next years to have another child were unsuccessful until my wife learned about an obstetric consultant who was trialling a surgical technique which introduced multiple stitches into the cervix to strengthen it sufficiently to carry babies to viability. Armed with the reassurance of joining the trial, my wife became pregnant in a further shake of a lamb's tail.

The programme required that she attended the hospital for weekly monitoring, which entailed a 200-mile round trip for her from our home every Monday morning. After just a few weeks of this, she was admitted for surgery and for the next 12 weeks or so she was bed bound in a city hundreds of miles from home, family and friends. Her sole purpose, day and night, was to wish her cervix back to competence.

We were communicating by phone, but her horizons were incredibly narrow, focussing on how to avoid pressure on the cervix – stay in bed – and on the regular but fearful measurements of its length. When calls were not made or not returned, I began to accustom myself to the idea of bad news. She was in a side room near the maternity ward and I began to feel a shameful hostility to all those expectant mothers and fathers who (with good reason) were discussing home births over water births, doulas over midwives, breast feeding and nannies; and wishing that they should share the horror of dead childbirth with us.

After one unreturned call, I tried to speak to but was unable to reach any member of the medical team – I had become inured to optimism and understood that something bad was underway. In a little while my foreboding was rewarded with the news that the pressure from our growing baby had been impossible to resist and that my wife had gone into labour, alone, that night. Our third baby, like his two brothers before him, had died in birth after being born too soon.

I had refused to believe that life would be so cruel to us (to anybody) as to prove that lightning could indeed strike the same place thrice. I was wrong. My wife, whose reaction was to harden into a fatalism about the inevitability of a life-long sadness, lost a precious hopefulness. The fissure in our relationship deepened into the Mariana Trench.

The inequity that I had a child and my wife was (and remained) childless appeared unbridgeable and was thus unspeakable. It was an imbalance that begged to be corrected. However, corrections of this sort and degree are inevitably painful. And five years after our third baby died, we divorced.

As you can see from mine and Declan's story, there were multiple other factors in the mix (he already had a child with someone else, I felt guilty about not getting our babies to term and out alive) that somehow stopped us from sharing our grief and, as we have seen, grief does not, in any event, march in a linear line whoever you are. Having thought so much, 30 years on, about the impact of a baby dying on both parents, I want to share this thoughtful comment made by a respondent to a recent Sands survey: 'Every individual person deals with grief differently. I don't like the stereotypes that come with a "men do this, women don't do that" kind of attitude. How we deal with grief depends on hundreds of factors, and only one of those is gender expectations.'

Joanna Froud, whose twin boys died within days of each other and shortly after their birth, is adamant that good therapy – finding a safe place to talk and, just as importantly, a good therapist who knows how to listen – saved both her, and her marriage to Matt.

As you read through her story below, you can pick out the slow shifts in the marriage that eventually helped this couple to reconnect and re-bond after the death of their baby boys. Saving the marriage took guts and determination from both parties but their story shows you can both change through your grief and still find each other again. (Matt tells his story on page 106.)

JOANNA'S STORY

It's 11 years since our twin boys died and I realise I now have a very different view. It happened, it was horrendous, but being a new Sands Befriender and listening to other people I realise just how far we have come.

How tricky it was – the dark days when you think you are never going to make it, and when you realise how many parents separate. It was tricky within the relationship and it was tricky with outside members of the family, but I am astounded by how it's changed my outlook on everything and how the experience of losing my two boys has formed me as a different person, for good and for bad.

I'm really talking about the immense joy of having gone through IVF again, of having had two further miscarriages but then of having got my two daughters. Don't get me wrong, I still shout at them like any normal mum, but every now and again, I'm stopped in my tracks and I think, 'Gosh, we did it. We found a happy place.' Which makes me so proud of all of us.

You've asked me how I found my way to this good place, 11 years on, and I have to say alcohol helped an awful lot; but, actually, we had hours of counselling with Child Bereavement UK, with a lady who hadn't lost a baby, and she was the making of us. Without her, we would have gone our separate ways. She just listened! She stopped us killing each other – she was bang in the middle, very non-judgemental – she cried with us a couple of times and she had us in separately a couple of times.

Every week we went. We wouldn't talk on the way there; we went through horrendous times. I wanted to cry and drink (self-medication and wanting to block the pain); Matt wanted to bury his head. After nine months, he went back to work; he threw himself into work and travelling and said he dreaded coming home to me.

So, the only thing we were really doing together was going to counselling, on the same day, every week. And afterwards we would go to the garden centre and have a toasted cheese sandwich. We would then talk in the garden centre; not for long but, after that, when he came home that night, things just felt easier. And so, bit by bit, I started to re-engage. I went back to my exercise class, although I didn't go back to hairdressing – my clients would have had no hair left!

The counsellor really was our saviour. So many of our friends who we thought were our friends weren't there for us – classic! And people we never imagined would be there for us came out of the woodwork and really supported us. We both changed, massively.

We had lost the boys in the April and, in the October, Matt said we need to go away. We booked an adults-only five-star resort in Turkey or somewhere and I remember being like a spoilt child telling my mum, 'I don't want to go. Look at my body . . .'

Anyway, we went on this holiday and it was almost like, now it's time to regroup.

We learned to laugh again, and cuddle, and it was like dating again. It was like being two new people because we had both changed so much; and letting him near me again was a big thing because I hated my body. I blamed my body for losing the boys. I hated everything. I hated my boobs. I hated the caesarean scar. Yet, when I look back now, I think, goodness, you looked good 11 years ago.

One night we went out and we got really quite merry and ended up in the nightclub at the resort where we made some really great new friends. We told those new friends about losing the boys and it felt like we were restarting us.

Anniversaries and such like are still difficult, but we've learned to come together and sensitively look after each other – we really have that depth in our relationship now. I am the luckiest, luckiest person to have kept him. And to have gone on to have our girls. We have a really solid relationship.

Then there is the impact on your relationship with your partner with all the IVF, the miscarriages and the surgeries. Plus, when we were going through all this, I had my father in a care home suffering from dementia telling me to 'pull my socks up'. They were tough, tough times. But I realise now we were so lucky we got to meet our boys, Joseph for just a week and Oliver for a month. That's a huge positive, although I know it's something the people who have a still-birth or a late miscarriage don't get. We were just so lucky to have had that.

Trying again was hard too. I always wanted to be a mum, right from being a little girl, and I wanted to fill that hole left by losing our boys, but Matt didn't really want to go through all that again and that felt like a divorce. My biological clock was ticking – I was 38 by the time we had our third child, my daughter Ellena, and 40 when I had her sister, Georgie, and, in the end, it was my mum who started to push, told me to get my skates on and keep going.

After we lost the boys it felt like Game Over. We took everything back to the shops and I remember rowing with John Lewis because I wanted to return the double pushchair; there was no point keeping it. We didn't have our children. And then, there was nothing; it was so quiet, so deathly quiet. I kept thinking, 'What am I going to do? Who am I?' So I felt I had no choice but to go again.

I have just become a Sands Befriender and when I sit with newly bereaved parents where the feelings are still so raw – that despair, that emptiness – it transports me right back. You know that they are sitting there thinking their lives are now over. But we are trained to listen; and maybe ask appropriate leading open questions to help them talk about those feelings if they want to.

Another thing that helps is having people who still acknowledge our boys. Every Christmas, my mother will put two stars on her card to us; she doesn't need to say anything because that speaks volumes. It's the quiet, little things like that which make all the difference. Now, if anyone has died, I go out of my way to remember to always bring that person up in a conversation.

I think it's going to take a long time to smash the taboo surrounding baby loss. With most people, the barriers go up; they think 'I am not going to acknowledge this because it's just too painful.' Sands is doing an amazing job, but it's still a huge mountain to climb and so we have no option but to keep talking, keep helping and do everything we can to bring the death rates down. I think we've got a long way to go but I really hope we do smash it.

A loss of any kind of sex drive is not uncommon after any pregnancy, let alone a pregnancy that ends in sorrow. Not only is the grief complicated, but feelings between you won't often be the same at the same time, which may have a hugely adverse impact on your physical relationship. You may now simply link the act of sex with the idea of creating a baby who then died which can trigger all kinds of anxieties about being intimate with your partner again.

Some couples may find sex comforting and reassuring after such a traumatic loss, but, as we saw in Joanna's story, bereaved mothers will often feel their body has 'let them down'. This will affect not only their self-esteem and self-worth but their desire to be sexual too. There may be changes to the body, including new scars, which can also impact on how a bereaved mother now feels about herself as a sexual being.

The important thing if any of this is happening to you is to try to just accept, rather than fight your feelings. They are your feelings for now. Don't try to be 'strong' and don't pressure yourself into doing anything you are not really ready for.

Physically healing from the birth of a baby takes around six weeks and, when grief and bereavement are in the mix, the psychological trauma may show up in physical difficulties including, for the woman, vaginal dryness and, for the man, difficulty having or maintaining an erection.

This is a complicated and distressing time so try to be patient with yourself and with each other. Perhaps accept, for now, that physical closeness like cuddling, hugs and holding hands is all you can manage and enough to keep the bond alive between you until you are ready to explore a sexual relationship together again.

If these issues persist and are troubling you, speak to a Sands counsellor or visit your family doctor and ask for a referral for psychosexual counselling.

CHAPTER 7

The Missing Sibling

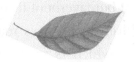

'A child who is old enough to love, is old enough to mourn.'

From 'Bereavement Reactions of Children',
KidsHealth, New Zealand

The impact of perinatal death on surviving siblings remains virtually unexplored. A child's understanding of death and its finality will depend on their age and emotional development, and if a dead baby is a challenge for adult grief, then all the more so for a child who is aware the baby – a potential brother or sister – has not come home; and equally so for those born into historical grief where the invisible presence of the older sibling will have already shaped the family narrative (see page 145 for more on this).

When a baby dies, your child will know you are intensely sad, and you cannot (and should not) try to hide your own grief from them. Instead, you need to understand the age-related broad guidelines regarding what a child may understand about death already and reassure them that what has happened – their brother or sister has died – is not their fault.

Children tend to grieve in bursts – sad one minute and back to playing the next. This does not mean the sadness has gone away; it hasn't, but younger children in particular will likely express their feelings of bereavement through behaviours, rather than words. And children of all ages may often seem entirely unaffected by the loss, which is misleading, because they *are* affected and, just as with adults, their grief can surface at odd times and resurface even years later.

Toddlers

Very young children have neither an understanding of death nor the language skills to express how they are feeling. They will know something bad has happened, picking up on the distress and anxiety of their parents, but their reaction will be a behavioural one. You may find them looking for the lost baby, crying more, being more clingy or being quieter and less responsive to you. The key to helping children of this age feel more safe and secure is to maintain normal routines and activities, hold and cuddle them more, keep the household as calm as you can and, if it feels right, give them a special comfort blanket or cuddly toy which, to your very young child, will feel reassuring.

'IN THE STARS'

In the Stars (published by Sands in February 2019) is a beautifully illustrated picture book, written by Sam Kitson and illustrated by her friend, Katie Faithfull, in memory of Sam's first daughter, Kitty, who was stillborn in 2009. It explores the death of a baby for younger children in a non-scary way based on the idea that, when we die, we return to nature and become part of its beauty.

Children process grief differently depending on their age, but questions you can expect from younger children, according to the book, include:

- Do you come back after you die?
- How can someone be in the stars, the trees and the flowers if they are in the ground?
- When are you going to die?
- When am I going to die?
- Why did another family's baby not die and ours did?
- Who will look after me when you die?

These are not easy questions for any parent to answer, never mind one grieving themselves but the goal, according to Sands, is to try to answer children's questions in as real and natural a way, by keeping your responses factual and simple; and, just as importantly, to understand that children move in and out of grief so that the question, 'When am I going to die?' may be followed by, 'What's for dinner?'

Sam says these are questions her own subsequent children, Martha and Amos, have asked her and that she and Katie were determined the book should be as beautiful as possible so that younger children would not be frightened by it.

KITTY: BORN 30 JULY 2009

We had had the perfect pregnancy with Kitty – no problems, no complications, I was healthy and loved every minute of it – and so we'd done it all; we knew we were having a girl, we'd chosen her name and prepared the nursery for her arrival so, when I look back, I can see we were way ahead of ourselves but you never expect this to happen to you.

One night, I realised Kitty had stopped moving. I had stomach cramps but wasn't in pain; I was 38 weeks into the pregnancy and so just thought I was in labour. Her dad, Woody, and I decided we'd go to hospital in the morning so we just went to bed that night.

The next day we went from all that happiness to the devastation of being told she had died, which you don't ever prepare for.

I'd been through bereavement before – I was very close to my grandparents and lost my granddad when I was 22 – but this was something else. Wood and I had only been together about two years when Kitty died, so I was really scared, after it all happened, that I would lose him, as well as her.

She was a planned baby because it had all felt so right; we'd got together pretty quickly, moved in together pretty quickly and I loved him. But we'd only been together a short time and so to go through something so horrendous together, I did feel like it was a make-or-break of our relationship. Neither of us knew how to deal with it. Neither of us had expected it; we'd been preparing for a birth.

We'd gone to the hospital that next morning, but they wouldn't let us see the screen at the scan. We were rushed off to another room where we were told Kitty had died. I remember them saying to me, 'Do you want to have her now?' I said, 'What? No! I want to go home.' I didn't want to be there – I needed some time to think about what was happening, so they gave me something to start labour and we went home for a day and two nights. That was very hard. I didn't want her to leave; I didn't want to have her, but I was struggling with knowing although I still had her here, she wasn't alive anymore. I just didn't want to let her go.

I found it so hard after Kitty died; I was really over-whelmed. I struggled over what had happened and Woody and I grieved very differently. My main thing was that I wanted to be happy and for us to still be together, so I worked really hard with a counsellor to try to make sure we would be OK. I loved Wood, and he'd been so amazing through it all, I didn't want us to then break up – that would have been a double whammy of hell.

Nobody was able to tell us why Kitty died. She had a post-mortem and we had her back a month after she had died so that we could have a funeral. That time gap was hard too because I was just ruminating on what I had done wrong to have caused this.

We'd gone back to the hospital and the consultant said: 'I can give you the best answer, you did nothing wrong.' But for me, that wasn't the best answer; it was the worst because I then spent years thinking, 'I killed her.' I'm sure he meant it was the best answer in order for me to go on and have other children – there were no genetic issues or placenta problems or problems with how my body had been in the pregnancy – but it's crazy to think, in this day and age, there are no answers to the question, 'Why did my baby die?'

I remember when we were burying Kitty and she was being lowered into the ground saying, involuntarily, to my mum: 'No, no . . . she can't go in there, she can't.' I just wanted to jump in there with her. I didn't want her to be down there in that ground. Wood had even asked at the hospital whether we could take her home and bury her in the garden. I know it sounds ridiculous, but we didn't want her to be anywhere else; we wanted her with us, whatever state she was in. She was our child. We wanted her home.

I felt I had failed Kitty; I had failed myself; I had failed my family. My one job was to get her here safely and I didn't do that. And I will never know why. Which is one of the hardest things to live with and, of course, it's one of the questions my subsequent kids, Martha and Amos, have asked a lot: 'Why did she die?'

The following January, just six months after Kitty died, I discovered I was pregnant with Martha. That was difficult too. I was so scared and although it felt right to be pregnant again, I felt guilty. The feelings were ridiculous; everything was so overwhelming but, through it all, it felt like there might be some light at the end of this horrific tunnel.

When I did come home with my second daughter, Martha, I just felt guilty. I'm loving another child, but it's not a replacement, and I don't want Kitty to feel like she's been replaced.

I kept a diary through Martha's pregnancy which I think

helped but I don't go back and read it anymore; it's just too painful. All the feelings are there; the guilt and the worry.

We didn't know we were having another girl; Wood had decided he didn't want to know the baby's gender because that would make it too personal. Which was really just a way of us trying to protect our feelings and distance ourselves from the pain should anything go wrong again, but, of course, you can't protect your feelings.

When Martha's head was delivered, she gave a strange little squawk and it was like she was reassuring me that she was alive. But even then, until I had her in my arms, I didn't believe there was going to be a live baby, at all.

When we brought Martha home, people would ask whether this was our first baby. And I would say no.

I feel really lucky I went on to have two healthy babies; we did think if it didn't happen, we might adopt but we were lucky. I only lost one baby. If it had happened again, I don't know if we would have carried on. I don't know how anyone survives multiple losses.

When you do come home with your baby, you have all those emotions of having a new baby living alongside your grief for your baby who died. It is a real mix of emotions. But I feel really lucky to have had two live kids; I always say that, and we still think that now.

And, sometimes, what happened with Kitty doesn't feel real anymore. I talk about it and it's as if it happened to someone else. I can reel off a load of facts to people, and timelines of what went on, and put myself back 'in there' for a second but I can't do it for very long because if I really think about it, it's too much and too painful.

While Sam sees the book as Kitty's legacy, it was also written because her other children, Martha, now ten, and Amos, eight, had, and still have, so many questions about the big sister they will never meet.

Sam, who had always wanted to write something in Kitty's memory, wrote the book one night in bed, and then Katie spent one-and-a-half years on the uplifting illustrations which support the idea that a baby who has died is still here; in the stars, in the flowers and all around.

The family had always had a picture of Kitty on the mantelpiece, so once the children started asking, she and Wood told them they had a big sister who had died. 'As the kids got older, they did start asking more questions, especially Martha,' says Sam. 'Although Amos is very sensitive and will get more upset and emotional when we talk about Kitty – and, of course, I don't want that – for Martha, who is closer in age to Kitty, the thought of having an older sister she will never know has been big for her.

'They both say they miss Kitty, but Martha will talk about what it would have been like to have a big sister and share a bedroom and what they would have been like together, wondering what they would have fought about, and whether they would have shared the same clothes.

'I have said to the children – you miss the idea of someone who hasn't been here and wasn't here when you were born, but they're the same kind of thoughts we've had as parents imagining that person who isn't here; what would she have been like now? Who would her friends have been? She'd have been going to high school this year . . . all those kinds of thoughts you have.

'But I have been very wary of and careful not to focus too

much on her dying and her death. I don't want their childhood to be about *Oh, Mum's sad because Kitty isn't here.* I've explained that she paved the way for them to be here and that there would never have been a time they'd have all been together because if Kitty had lived, they'd have been different babies.

'I wouldn't have had Martha so quickly, for example. It's hard trying to get that idea into my own head and then explaining it to them without it seeming scary. They have asked so many questions, including why she died. What happened? Did her heart just stop beating? Do lots of babies die? How did she get out; which meant we then had to talk a lot about birth.

'All of that ended up becoming part of the book. It's been really complicated with the kids to not force it upon them but then not forget Kitty either; that's been hard. It's a difficult path to navigate. Have I done it right? I don't know, but I would rather we talked about her and acknowledged her than it being some secret in the family.

'Wood's mum lost a baby years ago. She's been amazing and I think found it helpful talking to me about her baby who died who was called Emma. She hid that away for so long that Woods didn't even realise he'd had an older sister who had died until he was a lot older because, back then, it just wasn't talked about.

'Kitty is still our family and will always be our first baby, our firstborn, and I'd feel wrong to hide her away from the kids.'

(You can see Sam talking about the book, *In the Stars*, which is currently only available from the Sands shop, on a short video here: www.in-the-stars.co.uk/vids/ITS-intro-video.mp4.)

Pre-school Age

Children approaching school age will have some understanding of death – they will have seen films and cartoons where death features – but they are unlikely to really understand that death is permanent, and the dead baby will not be coming home, ever. This is a time of magical thinking in childhood so your child may believe if they wish hard enough or behave the best they can, the baby will come back to life and come home. They may also think the baby died because of something they did. Children in this age group will need a great deal of reassurance that the baby's death was not their fault and that you can, and will, keep them safe and looked after.

Tantrums and toileting problems are common behavioural signs of distress in this age group and, as before, they may go looking for the dead baby, have difficulty sleeping, dream of the lost sibling, show signs of being fearful and more anxious and even act out a regression in their own development by, for example, returning to crawling or asking for a bottle again.

Again, your job is one of maintaining normal routines and reassuring your child that they are safe and looked after. But with this age group, you can also help them find the right words for what they are feeling. You can say, 'I know you are feeling sad,' which teaches them this is the word for that feeling. Your physical presence will be important for your child at this time so try not to be apart for long periods. Cuddle and reassure them and perhaps explain that death is a part of life. Children at this developmental stage use play to explore the world and their feelings, so you can encourage this and even be a part of that play exploration.

'WHAT'S THE POINT, DAD?'

In Chapter 6, Sands United founder, Rob Allen, tells the story of how he hit on the idea of using football to connect grieving dads and give them a safe space to talk about their feelings.

Rob has a twelve-year-old son, Rhys, from another relationship and the couple share Alfie, now eight, who was just five when Niamh died. One of Rob's biggest fears was that Niamh's death would change Alfie, and that he would lose his innocence and some of his cheeky personality.

But while Alfie, says Rob, appeared to take Niamh's death in his stride having been told his baby sister was in heaven, he will still, from time to time, have what Rob calls 'a bit of a wobble' and surprise his parents with an astonishing question that puts them on the spot.

When he was seven, two years after his baby sister's death, he came down the stairs one evening after bedtime and said:

'I've been thinking . . . So, you're born, and the world spins round and round, and then you die. What's the point?'

'OK,' thought Rob. 'So, you're asking me existential questions at the age of seven and at half past eight at night. How do I answer this?'

In the end, he settled on explaining that during Alfie's 84-year-old grandfather's lifetime, lots of things had changed because people who had been born had invented many of the things that we all now take for granted. What that meant, he went on to explain to his young son, is that, really, we are all here to be the very best person we can be. He told his son that maybe he, Alfie, will grow up and invent something that helps people or become a doctor who finds the cure for a disease. He told his son all you have to do is find the thing that works for you.

'Oh, all right. OK,' Alfie replied, taking himself back off up the stairs to bed.

It seems Alfie was pretty satisfied with that answer, but it's probably fair to say that Rob and Charlotte are slightly dreading the next time they hear footsteps padding down the stairs with Alfie looking for the answer to another of life's big questions!

Primary School Age

Primary school children are still only starting to understand about death and may not yet understand that death is final. They may feel confused and worry that their dead sibling is lost and lonely and cold. Their questions may appear blunt and random. They may ask where the baby's body is and what happened. Explaining that death is final and that they don't have to worry about the dead baby's feelings is important in helping children of this age come to terms with their loss.

Behavioural changes you may see if your child is this age include (again) looking for the dead baby, dreaming of the dead baby and either becoming more clingy with you or more with-drawn. You may witness a sense of embarrassment – having a dead brother or sister means they are not the same as their school friends whose baby siblings did not die – and you may have to deal with physical manifestations of their distress, including tummy aches and headaches. They may not want to eat or go to bed at night. They may not want to leave your side and may show flashes of anger and antisocial behaviours.

You will need to reassure your school-age child in the same ways you would for younger children, but the big difference here is that you can – and should – involve your child more in the practicalities of the death, such as planning the funeral, and in any rituals you can share as a family to acknowledge the death of the baby and remember him or her (see Chapter 11). Again, encourage play, including drawing, writing and painting.

If you decide that a funeral is not the best way to help your child come to terms with the death of their sibling, there are other ways to have a goodbye. Planting a tree and sharing stories can all be good alternatives for providing closure to a child.

10–12 Years

If your child/children are older, in the 10–12-year age group, all the reassurance advice outlined above still applies, but, by this age, children understand that death is final. This age group will also be more acutely attuned to your own distress and grief and may ignore their own grief and feelings so as not to make yours worse. They may decide to be on their very best behaviour and try to take on more adult responsibilities so as to help and look after you. Children of this age will feel especially anxious about your safety, their own and that of family and friends. Death is now real. They too may blame themselves for what has happened, and you will likely witness stronger emotional reactions, including anger, guilt and a sense of rejection. Their questions may become incessant. They will be thinking a lot about their dead sibling and will want to talk about it.

As well as providing the reassurance they are loved, they are not to blame, they are safe and will be looked after, your key task with this age group is to acknowledge the depth of their feelings of grief and to be open and honest about what has happened and your own feelings. Because this age group will demonstrate grief and an understanding that death is final, you will also need to avoid having adult expectations of their grieving process, and of them, and remember they are still children trying to figure out what has happened and why it has happened to your family.

Teenagers

In a Swedish study of how adolescents reacted to the stillbirth of a baby, researchers reported teenagers having feelings of sadness and despair, injustice, helplessness, aggression and anxiety, much like their parents. And because balancing grief for a child who has died with caring for living children is difficult, adolescents taking part in this study noted that their parents were temporarily unavailable to them. Siblings then mourn both the loss of the baby and the loss of their previous relationship with their parents.

Teenagers know death is an integral part of life, but this may be their first personal experience of the grieving process. This means you may get reactions that fluctuate between the behavioural signs described for younger children and more adult expressions of their feelings of grief. Don't be hurt if your teen looks outside the family to talk about their feelings and find support. This is a pretty normal teen response to just about everything that happens in their life.

Your teenager may decide it's important to look as if they are coping well whereas, the truth is, they are struggling with the intensity of their grief. Signs of struggling can include an escalation of risk-taking behaviours to blot out feelings that threaten to overwhelm. Death can so disrupt a teenager that you may see more comfort-seeking behaviours with them turning to drink, drugs, more sexual contact or other reckless reactions. They may feel scared and unable to find the right words to express their difficult feelings. They may push you away, but inside they are hurting every bit as much as you.

Teenagers, just like younger children, may blame themselves for what has happened. Their performance at school may drop because of a difficulty in concentrating and you may find them unusually forgetful and distracted. A teen may start acting as if they don't care and may withdraw to avoid being close to others (someone else who might suddenly die). They may even use humour as a mask to keep their distance from you and from their grief and may end up feeling isolated, leading to depression and even suicidal thoughts. Make no mistake, a teenager's grief is every bit as complex and difficult to handle as an adult's and exacerbated by the sense they have lost the previous relationship they had with their parents – if only temporarily.

You will need to reassure your teenage child using all the parental skills you have at your disposal. Allow all their questions and answer them honestly. Involve them in funeral arrangements and remembrance rituals and make sure they know the grief they are feeling is normal but that everyone grieves in their own way so there is no right or wrong. Try to keep the household calm and loving, and show your teenager you are going nowhere and that they are safe and loved even though you too will be struggling with your own grief.

WHAT TO DO TO REASSURE A GRIEVING CHILD*

- Tell your child, whatever age they are, that they are safe and loved and looked after.
- Encourage age-appropriate talks about death and grief.
- Keep the household calm and be as honest and open with your child as you can be, and as their developmental stage allows.
- Try to maintain normal routines and activities.
- Give lots of reassurance.
- Tell your child that what has happened is not their fault.
- Be aware your living child/children may feel they have lost you and that you are no longer available to them. Make sure they know this is not the case. You are grieving but still there.

Bereaved parents, struggling with their own grief, may start to question their competence in parenting their living children, but it is worth remembering that your existing children will be invaluable to you in coping, as a family, with the aftermath of your terrible loss.

* Content and advice on helping grieving children is reproduced from KidsHealth (www.kidshealth.org.nz) with permission. KidsHealth content is endorsed by the Paediatric Society of New Zealand and supported by Starship Foundation and the Ministry of Health.

Historical Grief

Children born into a family following the death of a previous baby are born into something psychologists call 'historical grief'. They have no memory of a pregnancy, the expectation of a sibling coming home from the hospital or any first-hand experience of the grief throughout the family when that did not happen. But none of that makes the impact of grief in their childhood any less noteworthy. As stated at the start of this chapter, there is no research on the psychological impact of being born as a subsequent child into the family following a stillborn baby or neonatal death, although there has been some research into the bond between the mother and a subsequent child/children when a dead baby is part of the family history.

Erica Stewart, who tells the story of the death of her third child, Baby Shane, on page 88, did have another baby after Baby Shane and says she has often wondered about the impact on the only one of her children born into historical grief.

'The death of a baby does have an impact on a subsequent child,' she says. 'Some parents will idealise the baby that has died and, for the subsequent child, that can be a hard act to follow. They know the baby was special but sometimes the focus on that baby can leave a subsequent child feeling they are not as special. It's different with existing children because they were there and may even have met the baby, but for a child born after that death, what is the impact of visiting the grave or lighting a candle on their birthday?

'Parents have to be careful and try to find some kind of balance. I remember one parent telling me their two-year-old had picked up that the household was really sad and, for the child born subsequently, the parents now know the worst can happen and will be scared this child might die too for some reason. You know, when your baby has died, that your whole life can change in a second so you've always got that worry that your other children could die. If a baby can die, you now know anything can happen.'

Some researchers have explored the idea of a subsequent child born into the family after a baby dies as being at risk of 'replacement child syndrome' and suffering from the smothering over-attachment of an overprotective and fearful mother. But while there are earlier studies that supported this notion – notably one where the mother's perception of her child's overall difficulties and peer problems ranked higher among mothers who had suffered a stillbirth than those who had not – subsequent research has dismissed this idea finding no differentiated attitude between bereaved and non-bereaved mothers and thus denying the pathological existence of the 'replacement' or 'vulnerable' child.

Interestingly, there is no research whatsoever about the role fathers play when bereaved parents go on to have more children and must strike the balance between an understandable anxiety when a new baby is born, following the death of a baby born before them, and allowing their subsequent children to pass through the normal milestones of development and childhood.

The Blended Family

If there is a dearth of research into the impact of a baby dying on existing and subsequent children born into a family, there is no research at all into the impact of a baby death on the members of a blended family.

Jen Coates, Director of Bereavement Support and Volunteering at Sands, says: 'We need more work on the impact, depending on their age, on a sibling when they are bereaved through baby loss because, more and more, we have blended families and siblings who are therefore older when a baby dies.

'The complications of a stepfamily, and the place of the children within it, when overlaid with bereavement over a baby they may have had very mixed feelings about in the first place, is an area we really need to look at because we know that within a blended family this type of bereavement may sit in a different place.

'In any family, when a baby has died, children who follow on may ask themselves whether they would even have existed if that hadn't happened. Or perhaps that's a question parents ask themselves. It may not occur to a child to ask themselves that, or maybe not until they are adults when they can explore it, but the truth is, while we know a baby death has an enormous impact on children of the family, we just don't know the extent of that impact.'

CHAPTER 8

Everyone
Else . . .

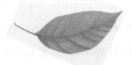

'The process of grieving can feel wild and nonlinear
– and often lasts for much longer than other
people, the nonbereaved, tell us it should.'

Jeffrey Rubin, from *Bearing the Unbearable*
by Joanne Cacciatore

When a baby dies there is the terrible grief of the parents, but
it will affect – even shock – everyone who comes into contact
with the intense pain and sorrow that follows. It is as if a pebble
shatters the surface of a pool of water spreading ripples to the
edge. For every one of the 14 babies who die every day in the
UK, the number of other lives changed forever is considerable.

In this chapter we explore the impact on the people who love the parents and want to support them.

The Sister

Every morning, a mum of five gets off the tube at King's Cross station in London, picks up a Santander bike outside the station and cycles for half an hour to reach the Victoria offices of the charity where she has worked for the last three-and-a-half years. At the end of the day, she pedals back using the time, and the mindless pedalling, to think about everything and nothing.

That woman is Clea Harmer, the CEO of Sands.

CLEA'S STORY

As a junior doctor, I did paediatrics but that was at a time – the late eighties – when there wasn't much understanding of the impact of baby death and, sadly, from the point of view of many healthcare professionals, it was often 'just one of those things'. There wasn't really a feeling that anything could be done about it. I remember being very upset by this as a junior doctor; seeing the numb devastation on the bereaved parents' faces and the total inability of some of the healthcare professionals to reach out to them. The parents seemed to be so on their own and so isolated.

My first exposure to baby death was the death of a tiny baby – a neonatal death. Back then the NICU – neonatal intensive care unit – was nothing like it is now, so sadly often not a lot could be done for these tiny babies. You don't ever forget the babies who die when you are a doctor; you remember each one very specially.

When I had my own first child, I moved out of medicine and into editing medical publications and was then drawn into antenatal education. A lot of what I was doing was around education for pregnancy and early parenting. It is so important to introduce the idea of loss in antenatal classes, but so often it doesn't happen because it just feels 'too difficult'. We must help break the silence about baby death in antenatal classes so that parents know it is a possibility, and so that others in the class can help by reaching out to support parents if their baby does die.

Underpinning everything, and more important than anything, is the death of Clement, my nephew.

My sister is only 15 months younger than me, so we have always been very close. I'd had my first baby and we were then pregnant together. My sister was expecting her first baby and I was expecting my second; she was due in July and I was due in December. Clement was very overdue and, looking back, I should have been encouraging my sister to go in to be induced, but instead I reassured her that everything would be fine. It wasn't fine; Clement died during labour.

The grief and the guilt that I feel are so closely entwined; the deep, deep sadness of not having Clement, but also the overwhelming and almost physical feelings of pain and grief for my sister. Her beautiful son lying so very still in her arms, she looked literally crushed – and there was nothing I could do to change anything. I thought I could make the physical ache for her and for Clement in some way better by 'sharing' my baby when he was born – but it didn't, of course it didn't.

I couldn't take the pain away, but I could try and walk beside her in her grief – at times that has felt utterly inadequate, but it is a journey that I feel privileged to have been on.

It is an extraordinary honour to be the CEO of Sands – it feels as if I have been given a unique and very special opportunity to do something for Clement and to make a difference.

I have learned an enormous amount from everyone I have met and worked with. I have learned about unimaginable grief, about loneliness and isolation, and about anger and sadness; but I have also learned about resilience, about generosity and kindness, and about courage and love. I know I have been changed, I have understood so much more about my own journey, and I have been humbled by the journey of others. I just hope it means that I can use all my experiences to make things better for others in a way that I couldn't for Clement and my sister.

Clea started in the role of CEO of Sands on 25 July 2016. She had been asked to start at the beginning of the month but asked if she could delay until the twenty-fifth, which would have been her nephew Clement's twenty-fifth birthday.

The Grandmother

Gerry Ward, who celebrates her eightieth birthday this year, is mum to Joanna Froud, who talks about the difficult emotions she faced after the death of her twin boys on page 123 and mother-in-law to Joanna's husband, Matt, who describes the birth and death of those children in Chapter 6.

Here is what Gerry has to say about the impact when your child's baby or babies die:

We were told, but we didn't understand at the time, that there can be huge problems with multiple births and identical twins. They did try to warn us, but I looked at Jo and Matt, who were both the picture of health and happiness, and couldn't imagine anything going wrong.

The pregnancy was being filmed by a TV programme being made about identical twins and we were excited to be involved with that; it was something different and they were following Jo through the pregnancy coming to each scan and talking to her after each appointment with the consultant. After the boys died, we never heard from them again.

When the twins were born by caesarean at 30 weeks and 3 days, they were very tiny, and I remember going up in the lift to intensive care with one of them. He was so tiny and there was a crowd of doctors going up in the lift with us, but nobody said anything. The second twin soon followed so then they were both in intensive care. We knew they were poorly; they were very, very poorly.

A few days later, the consultant asked to speak to us in a side room and told us they didn't think one of the twins, Joseph, was going to live and so asked if we would like a photo. I remember thinking, 'Good God, no. . .', but I was wrong, because since then, we've often looked at the photos of the boys and she was right, having photos has been important to us.

Joanna came home after Joseph died, and we would go to the hospital and sit for hours and hours with Oliver, the surviving twin. We'd go home and all the congratulations cards and presents were flooding in, as they do, and at the same time, all the sympathy cards arrived saying we are sorry Joseph has died.

You just feel, what can I do? Matt, who I am so fond of, is lovely but he didn't want to talk about it whereas Jo desperately needed to talk about it. We went over and over everything. I just felt so helpless, not knowing how I could help them both. I was utterly bereft. It was absolutely awful seeing my own child in that much pain – sobbing and sobbing – and knowing I couldn't do anything about it and yet, as the mother, you think you should be able to do something.

On the evening of Joseph's funeral, the hospital called to say Oliver had taken a turn for the worst. He also had the same gut infection as his brother. We all rushed back to the hospital, where he died 18 hours later; it was just awful. Jo was desolate when her second baby died – she was angry and couldn't understand why this had happened to her.

I don't think unless you have been through this experience, anyone can really understand. All the hours we had spent sitting in intensive care and, of course, hearing everybody else's problems because you all get to know each other. When people say they've lost a baby and other people say, 'Oh dear, that's sad . . .' – the truth is that it is much, much more than that.

I didn't have anyone I could talk to through it all. My husband was in a nursing home with Alzheimer's. He was the loveliest man you could wish to meet, very kind, very considerate, but he just said to Jo, 'Pull yourself together,' which nearly killed her. He couldn't help it.

I have a sister and I have a lot of friends, but they don't understand. I don't say that unkindly, because I know that when I now hear about someone having these kinds of problems I understand much more. I don't think you can expect other people to know the pain unless they have gone through it too.

Sometimes I knew Joanna needed space, but it was difficult to know when to leave her and when to stay with her. I'd be driving home wondering whether I was right to leave her because, often, she didn't know what she wanted from me.

I find it difficult too, with each year that passes, to know what to do on the anniversaries of the boys' deaths. We talk about the boys, but I am quite guarded because her two girls who were born after the boys died are still quite young and I do wonder if they are frightened that they might die too.

There are so many difficult things. If Joanna goes for an appointment and the doctor or someone asks how many children she has and she says, 'I had four, but I lost two,' nobody says, 'Oh, I'm so sorry,' they just say, 'Right . . .' and move on. When she tells me this, I think, 'Oh, come on, just acknowledge them.' Doctors should know better!

I think all bereaved parents are asking for it to be acknowledged that they had these children. People don't understand either that it take a lot of guts to have another baby after this. I wanted Joanna to try again and pushed her. She was a broken woman. Matt didn't want to try again because he was frightened, but I knew that all Joanna wanted was to have a little family, so I think I probably did more than pushing.

155

I felt very strongly that's what they needed. I found myself in the situation many times after the boys died, and I'm sure other family members of people who have lost a baby will have done this, where we'd go out and I'd have to make sure we were sitting somewhere where there weren't other children or families around.

I know the grief of losing their boys will never, ever leave them, but Jo and Matt have swum back up and I am incredibly proud of them. She's out there; onwards and upwards, helping with Sands and wanting to do counselling now because without counselling I think they would have grown apart because they couldn't talk about it together.

When Jo asked me if I would contribute to this book, I wondered why. But then I understood that as someone's mum you have a big role to play, not in their recovery, but in your child coming to terms with the cruelty of life when this happens.

'Most mothers found it very difficult to be in situations that reminded them of "what could have been." Examples of these situations were being around pregnant women or infants, attending baby showers, and celebrating holidays.'

From the 2018 *Lancet* series on stillbirth

The Best Friend

I'm not sure if I can imagine a harder road ahead than the one facing the best friend of a mother whose baby has died and whose first response, naturally, to the shock and trauma of that experience may be to disappear behind an almost impenetrable wall of 'radio silence'. When you are the best friend, although you will have your own feelings of shock and grief to deal with, you will want to park those so that you can support your friend even when you (and they) have absolutely no idea how best to do that.

What do you do or say when you hear the shattering news that your friend has come home to an empty nursery and a life changed forever by their sadness and loss? How will you cope with your own feelings of guilt if you did come home with your baby and if those children, which is likely when your friendship is age-matched, would have been close in age? How will you know how much or how little to say about your own family life and your own children (if you have any) or how much of the outside world to take into the home of your bereaved friend, assuming you can get through the front door to see them?

Let's start with that assumption – that you will be able to see your friend – because the likelihood is, until they can start to make some sense of this new 'unreality' and unexpected narrative to their life, they probably won't want to see you or anyone else. It's just too hard.

WhatsApp and text messages may, at first, go unanswered; voicemails and emails the same. It will be hard for you to resist the feeling that you are being rejected – mainly because you *are* being rejected, but only as part of a rejection of everything that was previously 'the norm', so your first task will be to develop a thicker skin and not take those rejections personally.

Your second task, especially if your bereaved friend has shut the door on the outside world for now, will be to keep knocking at that door – the literal and metaphorical barrier currently preventing you from connecting – and just keep knocking until you can find your way in. There may, at some point, be a need for some indelicate 'barging' in because, for some, this is not a door that is going to open easily to very many people outside the inner sanctum of the couple who have lost their child.

If you have experienced grief in your own life then you already have the starter tools for the difficult job ahead of supporting your friend, avoiding saying the wrong things and trying to understand their rage and bitterness which may, in some unspoken way, end up being directed at you, especially if you got to bring your own baby home.

There are ways you can support your friend when their baby dies, starting with practical support and taking over the things that will help shield them as they process the early stages of their grief – you can do all the things suggested here, and more, but only if your friend allows you to.

In the early days and weeks after their baby dies, many bereaved parents find it extremely difficult to do everyday things, such as cooking, housework, shopping, sorting out bills or walking the dog. Parents may find it useful if you are able to offer to help with some of these things but be aware that they will also need privacy sometimes, even if they want you to be around at other times. And sometimes, as Gerry noticed with her daughter Joanna, they won't know what they want from you. So, it may be helpful if you offer to leave after providing some help. On the other hand, if they need you to stay for a while and you know you have only limited time, it is best to let them know this early on in the visit.

Nine years ago, Sam O'Reilly threw a baby shower for her

best friend who was due to give birth to her first child in the January, after the Christmas holidays. New mum Sam, who had given birth to her second daughter just four months before, was concerned when her pregnant friend arrived feeling anxious about the size of her baby bump and seemed to be not her usual exuberant and confident self.

'I watched her opening the baby shower presents and while she was thanking everyone and saying how pleased she was, I could tell there was something. She just seemed quiet,' Sam recalls. 'She had asked me, when she arrived a couple of days earlier and we had gone out for lunch, if I thought her bump was small for her stage of pregnancy and I had suggested we could go to hospital and have it checked, but she said her mum had told her that her pregnancies had been small and that, in any event, she had a midwife appointment booked for when she returned home a couple of days later.'

The friends parted after the baby shower and Sam was pleased and relieved when her friend rang to say all was well; she had heard the baby's heartbeat and the midwife had said, 'This is a textbook pregnancy.'

A few days passed and Sam realised that none of her text messages were being returned when she'd messaged to check on her best friend. Her follow-up phone calls too had remained unanswered.

'I knew, I just knew there was something wrong,' she recalls. 'There was just this awful radio silence.'

A few days later, Sam's best friend's husband rang her to tell her the couple's baby had died.

'He was very, very upset and so it was a very short phone call,' says Sam, who cries again as she remembers that devastating call. 'We were both sobbing. I was in shock, obviously, and just kept saying, "I'm sorry, I'm so sorry."

'I asked what I could do, but he didn't really say anything. He was just too upset. After the call, I sent my friend a message but there was no contact back. In fact, there was no contact for quite some time. I felt really upset and really helpless and sad. We live in different parts of the country, so the distance was a problem, plus I was still on maternity leave with a small baby myself.

'I felt desperate to get to her, but I couldn't drive at the time which didn't help. I couldn't get to her, but I knew that she didn't want to see me anyway. She was too broken. I felt frustrated, desperate, sad and incredibly guilty because her baby girl had died, and I had two daughters who had lived.

'I think that was quite a big thing in our friendship because after her baby had died all she yearned for was a daughter and I had mine. That was really hard for me. And so, although we were speaking, it was still a good couple of months before I actually saw my friend.'

Eventually, Sam says she almost had to just turn up on the doorstep. The friends had been text messaging a bit but whenever they had tried to speak on the phone, both of them had just cried.

'There were no words,' says Sam. 'There was nothing I could say. But I knew that for the very first time in her life, she was well and truly broken. Until this, nothing bad had ever happened to her and I felt like this – her baby dying and grief on this scale – was just too big to handle.

'When she opened the door to me it was incredibly emotional. We cried and cried and cried and I kind of didn't recognise her. She looked – and this is the only way I can describe how she looked – absolutely broken. She was trying to keep her mind busy; I remember she was doing a tapestry, but the emotion was just pure grief and disbelief and sadness.'

The emotion that followed those initial feelings of devastation was anger, says Sam, and, for the best friend, this can be one of the hardest reactions to witness and know how to deal with.

In the end Sam dug deep into the resilience toolbox and took out the one tool that was going to allow their long friendship to survive and even grow past the trauma and the grief of the baby having died.

'In the end, I just listened,' she says.

'I listened, and I listened, and I listened. Because I needed her to know that I was supportive.'

During our conversation about how best to be a best friend to someone whose baby has died, I edge into the difficult territory with Sam of how she managed to talk about her own daughters through the early stages of the shattering grief she witnessed her friend struggling with.

'I didn't,' she told me. 'I just didn't really talk about them.'

Sam says her bereaved friend would ask after her girls and that today, almost a decade on from the death of her own baby daughter, she loves Sam's girls and is as involved with their lives as she is with the lives of the two subsequent children she went on to have. But back in those early stages of grief, neither of the two friends could face that yawning gulf between them: one friend raising her two young daughters, one struggling to understand how and why hers wasn't with her because she had died.

Back then, when the friends did spend time together, Sam would always turn up on her own, as the best friend and not with her own family in tow.

'I don't think we got together again as two families until she had her second child,' she says. 'It wasn't so much I felt like we couldn't do it before then, it was just easier for me to see her alone because my work meant I was away from my family sometimes and when I was, I would stay with her. But the truth is, although all that made sense back then, I just felt too guilty about having my daughters when she had lost hers.'

Grief, as we have seen, is not a linear challenge. A good day may be followed by three days right back to the pain and anger of the beginning which means a good friend is going to have to 'read' the situation and work out what kind of support, if any, is needed.

'I think I did that bit quite well because I know my friend so well,' says Sam. 'I also started to get angry myself when I saw how some of her other friends started to distance themselves. She lost some very close friends simply because they didn't know how to deal with it.'

I have yet to meet a bereaved mother (or father too) who has not experienced the 'disappearing friends act' that so frequently and swiftly follows the death of a baby. Those are the friendships that will never get back on track but this is not an option for you because you are The Best Friend and this couple has already lost so much; your continued involvement, albeit dictated by them as to how much involvement and in what ways, will mean everything to the family as they slowly start to grow around their grief. Slowly. Painfully slowly, which means you might want to pack your 'support' toolbox with endless layers of super-human patience.

Think of it this way. There's been a fierce storm; a tempest that has raged through the hopes and very identity of these parents. The damage has been monumental. Hope and love and all the other good stuff are out of sight for now. Not gone, well, not for good, but not accessible when this first happens and, frequently, for a long time after. Hopefully, you can draw on empathy (you know sympathy is not what's needed) and you may even be very good at imagining the terrible pain your best friend is now in, but there is a huge barrier that you will both need to fight to overcome because, however empathic you are, this did not happen to you. It happened to her. And him. And the baby they thought they would be bringing home.

There are no social niceties that can help you tolerate this onslaught of fury, shame, guilt, sorrow and yearning to turn back time. You are going to have to turn up, stripped bare of any of the normal strategies we all use to nurture and navigate our relationships, and just make it clear, by your presence and willingness to get tossed around by the tempest, that you love your friend and you're not going anywhere; no matter how hard it gets or what you then have to do to cope with the fallout from the storm which will not leave you – or anyone in its wake – miraculously undamaged.

As you prepare to show up and offer your loving support, you will need to make sure the toolbox you are filling is made of resilience. Because you're going to need it, and not just for a week or two, or even a few months. You are going to need it for the rest of the entwined lives you've shared and want to continue to share.

When asked how it was that she, Sam, could tolerate her friend's intense grief, her reply is unhesitant: 'I love her. We'd already been through a lot together and we know each other so well. I could see the pain in her, I could see how broken she was, and I just couldn't understand why that wasn't visible to other people.

'Maybe it was because I had just had a child myself, and so I could put myself in her shoes and I could understand the pain she was going through. I don't know whether I could have done that if I hadn't had two daughters myself, but I just kept putting myself in her position, all the time.'

I think what Sam has just talked about is empathy. She was not afraid to sit with her grieving friend; putting her own life on hold when she could so that she could hold her heartbroken friend's hand and listen, quietly and carefully, to whatever she needed to say.

THE ANTENATAL GROUP

Several of the bereaved mums who shared their stories with me winced when they spoke about 'being the only one' in the antenatal class who did not come home with a baby and admitted that, for the most part, it was just easier to let those newly-formed relationships slide now the common bond – a baby – was no longer shared.

Taking the path of least resistance is understandable but some of the mums were also hurt that nobody from the class contacted them after their baby died to say how sorry they were, which tells us that even when you come home from hospital without your baby, having that loss acknowledged by those with whom you did share some of the happier early months of pregnancy feels important.

The onus here is not on the bereaved mother to initiate the first move. The onus is on those members of the group who felt close to her to let her know how sorry they are and how they are thinking about her and the baby who died. There is nothing more to say and, although it may not seem much, it will mean a lot to the grieving parents that you found the courage to let them know they are in your thoughts. And if you are still pregnant and awaiting the birth of your own child, it will take courage to put your own feelings of fear – it is so scary to think that this could happen to you – to one side to let a bereaved family know you are thinking of them.

How Best to Support Newly Bereaved Parents

When a baby dies in utero, parents are usually offered a number of choices about how they would like to give birth and what they might want and need in terms of making memories and spending time with their baby. There are no right and wrong decisions and parents need to decide what is best for them. Depending on the situation, you may also find yourself being invited to be involved. It is important to try to take your cue from the parents rather than imposing your views or needs on to them.

If a baby is stillborn or has died shortly after birth, parents are asked if they would like to see and hold their baby and, for many parents, this time spent bonding with their baby becomes a precious memory. Not all parents will decide to see their baby, but, if they do, the parents may then ask if you would like to see and hold the baby too. If they do, and you feel this is something you would like to do, you will find that seeing the baby can give you precious memories to share with the parents in the future. It can also be helpful for parents if someone else has seen and perhaps held their baby. If, however, the parents invite you to see or hold the baby, and you do not feel able to do so, it is important to be honest and let the parents know in as gentle a way as possible that this is not something you feel able to do and share with them.

Parents may also want to create memories of their baby and, depending on what they decide, you may also want to ask about creating your own keepsakes. If, for example, the parents decide to have photos taken, these photos may include some of the baby alone, with one or both parents, with brothers and sisters, or with you or other family members. You may then want a photo to keep and perhaps display in your home.

If the parents have named the baby, and they would like people to use the baby's name, it is important that you do this as well. Using the baby's name is an important acknowledgement for many parents. You may also want to include the baby when talking about how many grandchildren, cousins, nieces or nephews you have, but ask what the parents would like you to do.

Never impose what you think is needed or most helpful on the grieving parents but take your lead from them. One common mistake is family or friends thinking they are being thoughtful and acting for the best by removing any signs of 'baby' including baby equipment and clothes before a couple comes home from the hospital. Don't do this, because, however well-intentioned, it will likely backfire. What you can do is sensitively check whether this would actually be helpful. Many parents prefer to clear away the baby's things themselves in their own time, even though it may be weeks or months before they feel able to do so. Doing this in stages might help them with the grieving process and it is very important not to rush the parents into getting rid of or donating things that they might have had ready for the baby.

Depending on the baby's gestational age at delivery and on the parents' preferences, there may be a funeral. How will you cope if you are invited to attend? You may be asked to give a reading or even be godmother or godfather to a baby you never met and will never know. Could you do that for your friend or family member? Or it may be the case, which it often is, that the parents don't want anyone else (including you) at the funeral. Or that they may not even have a service. This can be hard too because you will have also invested in the baby that should have come home and so will likely be suffering a bereavement, the extent of which may have shocked you. If this is the case, then you need to find someone to talk to about your grief (see below).

It is important to listen to the parents to understand what support they need. Everyone grieves differently, so offering a form of help that might have been beneficial for you in the same situation might not be helpful for them. If they refuse your offers of help or want to be alone, you may feel hurt or excluded. However, they need to do what feels right for them at the time. This does not mean that they will not value further efforts you may make to support them when they are ready. They may also be so distressed that they cannot appreciate your offers of help.

It can be very difficult to find the right balance between being supportive and being intrusive. It can also be hard to show bereaved parents that you care without saddening them with your own grief, making them feel that they need to support you, or that your grief 'overshadows' theirs. They may need to be reassured that you care about their baby and about them; however, if there is one thing that is more important than any other guidance for family and friends, it is that bereaved parents should not feel that they have to comfort you.

Relationships can come under additional strain when there is a bereavement, and grief may make it harder than usual to see other people's points of view and to accept different ways of doing things. It can be helpful to remember that remarks about how you think the parents are coping, or advice on how you think they should be grieving, can feel hurtful. Being there to listen is often the best form of support.

In addition to providing support to the parents, you might find that you grieve together. This could be helpful as long as each person is doing what they need at the time. It can be useful, too, to allow time to grieve separately.

SYLVIE'S POEM

Thoughts consumed by thoughts of you and
the devastation you must feel.
I can't imagine what you're going through,
I only wish that it weren't real.
But where there is light,

> there is hope and there will always be light.
> You just have to hold your head high and
> stay brave throughout the night.
>
> In the meantime, look to the sky,
> take the star that your eyes first chose,
> and there, helping light up the night sky,
> is your beautiful Sylvie-Rose.
>
> By Aaron Bird, uncle to Sylvie-Rose, 2013

The above poem was written by a grieving uncle to the niece he would not get to see grow to adulthood. However, it isn't just immediate family and friends who will be affected when a baby dies. The neighbour on the opposite side of the street may not be a friend but will have seen a baby bump and wonder what happened when the house suddenly becomes shrouded in what looks to an outsider like a mysterious silence. The person serving at the corner shop who may have asked about the baby every time Mum popped in for a pint of milk will find it hard not to react when the next time they see her she is without a bump and without a baby.

All these causal encounters that make up the tapestry of our lives will have to be handled and, again, this is something the extended family or best friend can do for a bereaved couple; explain that the baby died and that when their paths cross with those of the bereaved parents again, the best response is the simplest one which is just to say, 'I am so sorry your baby died.'

BEING AROUND OTHER BABIES

Many bereaved parents won't want to say so, but they will find it distressing to be around other expectant or new parents and babies, which can be very hard on any family member or friend who is still pregnant or has a healthy baby. It can be especially difficult for the parents of a new-born baby in the family or a couple's social circle who may feel constrained and unable to celebrate their baby's arrival as they would like. It is important to recognise and acknowledge this and maybe give bereaved parents a private opportunity to meet the new baby when they are ready.

> - If there are existing children in the family, offer to take over the school run and the logistics for extra-curricular activities.
> - Check if you can help with cooking or shopping.
> - Offer to let the wider friendship group know what has happened and what your friend's preferences are with regards to condolences, cards and flowers, etc.
> - Act as the go-between if there is a funeral that people other than the immediate family can attend.
> - Offer to walk the dog, take the cat to the vet or do any of those extra tasks that may feel overwhelming for a newly bereaved parent.
> - Encourage the parents to talk about what happened at the hospital, the time they spent bonding with their baby and all the feelings, including the horrible ones, that have followed since coming home without their child.

Coping With Your Own Grief and Feelings of Loss

The death of a baby at any time during pregnancy is a major bereavement for the baby's parents. However, how the death affects the wider family isn't often fully understood or acknowledged. Not everyone realises the need for other family members or close friends to grieve or to share their distress and, because this need is so poorly understood, family and friends themselves may be taken aback, at first, by the intensity of their own grief.

It is possible that you might grieve both for the loss of the baby and for the loss of your own hopes and dreams. You may also grieve for the parents too. It can be extremely upsetting to see someone close to you in distress and be unable to protect them or to take their pain away. If you are a relative, you may also experience difficult feelings of guilt if the baby had a hereditary condition, even though there was nothing anyone could have done to prevent it.

For some relatives and friends, the death of the baby might also bring back painful memories of their own experience of having had a baby who died. Until the 1980s, the death of a baby was often not recognised as traumatic and most parents did not receive much understanding or support. Parents were likely to have been told to forget about their baby, to have another, and to carry on as though nothing had happened. They may not have been allowed to see or hold their baby or make any special memories. However, even with sensitive and supportive care, the grief that follows a baby's death remains and may be reawakened many years later.

It is normal for those trying to support and care for someone whose baby has died to experience strong emotions of sadness and loss themselves. If this is happening to you, you are also very welcome to access Sands' support resources and the Sands helpline, and if you are finding it hard to manage everyday life or work, you may want to seek professional help. You can make an appointment with your GP and explain how you are feeling. They can refer you for specialist help and support if needed. You may also like to seek counselling directly. If you are feeling overwhelmed and surprised by this sadness, then please do get in touch with the Sands bereavement team to help you with this.

CHAPTER 9

Returning to Work

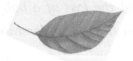

'There were a few people at work who just never spoke to me again . . . I mean I definitely got the feeling . . . like I was bad luck.'

Bereaved mum

According to a recent Sands survey, almost half of all bereaved parents reported that nobody said a word to them about their dead baby when they returned to work. Not one word. Not surprisingly then, about the same number said they did not feel supported in returning to their role in the workplace and that even when there was some kind of acknowledgement or communication, four in ten employees described those communications as being neither 'sensitive' nor 'appropriate'.

Half of employers, according to the survey, failed to provide any information on entitlements to pay and leave following the death of a baby so again, not surprisingly, only one in five of those surveyed were aware of their employer's bereavement policy – or even whether they had one.

A new Parliamentary Act introduced in January 2020 makes it now a legal requirement in the UK for employers to provide a minimum of two weeks' paid leave for any employee, male or female, whose baby or child has died.

'Returning to work after the loss of a baby is isolating and overwhelming. Training staff to understand how they can support colleagues after such a devastating loss will help make that step a little less daunting.'

Emma Cann, Framework Lead, Lendlease

Sands staffer, Ross Jones, is part of the Improving Bereavement Care team and works with a special focus on helping educate employers and HR teams to better understand the impact on a parent/employee when a baby dies, and to have the confidence to better know what to say when that employee returns to work.

A year ago, in collaboration with Lendlease, Sands launched a pilot scheme offering employer workshop training days exploring how best and better to welcome a bereaved parent back into the workplace and, crucially, how to avoid that parent feeling increasingly isolated when colleagues opt to avoid them rather than do or say 'the wrong thing'.

'When an employee has a baby it's not unusual for their workplace to send cards or flowers or a gift, but when a baby dies, most bereaved parents will hear nothing,' says Ross. 'That can be the start of an increasingly isolating experience of the workplace after your baby has died and came up quite a lot in our "Finding the Words" surveys.

'Nobody wants to be insensitive deliberately, but what a lot of employers struggle with is communication around the time of bereavement; what should they do or say when they learn that an employee's baby has died? Another challenge for employers and other employees is lack of awareness and knowledge about the impact on an employee of the death of their baby.

'People at work don't want to make the situation any more painful than it already is; they just can't imagine what it must be like when your baby dies and don't know what to say or do; they worry they might make things worse by saying or doing the wrong thing so they will often choose, instead, to say nothing. Also, employers may not have communicated what their policies are and this can leave bereaved parents making not good choices at such a difficult time. They don't know their rights.

'What I've seen, working at Sands over the last five years, is the charity acting almost as a bridge in that way, bringing the voices and experiences of the bereaved families to working closely with professionals and making sure they work together to improve systems and services. I think it's something quite unique.'

'Work incorrectly marked me as sick instead of on maternity leave and I had to get that changed retrospectively.'

Marie Farrelly, bereaved mum

If, like Marie above, you were working before your baby was born, you may be starting to think about going back to work.

For some bereaved parents, the idea of returning to a work routine can feel helpful, while for others the whole idea of returning to work may feel and turn out to be very daunting. The decision about when to go back to work will depend on how you are feeling; your physical and emotional health; and also your finances and perhaps other work-related factors. The first step needed to make an informed decision is to know your legal rights.

If you are the birth mother, your baby died either before or during birth, and your baby was at least at 24 weeks' gestation, this is considered a stillbirth in law and you are entitled to the same leave as mothers in your position whose babies are born alive. This could include Statutory Maternity Pay (SMP), Maternity Allowance or income-related benefits from the state. The same entitlements apply if your baby was born alive and then died, even if your baby was born before 24 weeks' gestation. If these rights apply to you then you may feel you don't need to think about returning to work for some time.

If you are self-employed, you are not entitled to SMP. However, depending on how long you have been self-employed and what National Insurance contributions you have made, you may be entitled to Maternity Allowance.

If you are a partner, or a co-mother, you are entitled to one or two weeks of parental or paternity leave. Couples can also take Shared Parental Leave as long as notice to take the leave was given before the baby died.

Unfortunately, if your baby died before birth and was under 24 weeks' gestation, this is considered a late miscarriage and so you are not entitled to maternity leave or maternity allowance. However, birth mothers who have early or late miscarriages may be entitled to sick leave as long as their GP can provide a note to this effect.

It is good practice for your employer to record sickness following miscarriage separately from other sick leave so that it does not count towards your sickness record. Long-term sickness could form part of your sickness record.

Compassionate leave may be granted for bereaved parents, but this will be at the discretion of the employer.

The Parental Bereavement (Leave and Pay) Act came into effect in 2020 and requires employers to offer an additional two weeks of paid leave to anyone who experiences the death of a child under the age of 18. This entitlement does not depend on the length of service. Parents of babies who are stillborn are also entitled to this leave. The leave will need to be taken within 56 days of the bereavement, although it does not have to be taken as block leave. And Parental Bereavement Leave is independent of maternity leave.

When you are ready to think about going back to work, you need to contact your employer to discuss practical details. You may be offered, or want to request, a phased return to work. This could involve working only a few days a week or a few hours each day for the whole week.

You could also explore the option of working from home or flexible working. If you have a full-time job, you could also request part-time working for a short period of time. Although employers have a legal obligation to consider this, there is no legal obligation for them to accept the request.

Once you have agreed a date to return to work, you may find it helpful to talk to your manager or employer about how you are feeling and what might help you settle into the work environment.

You could also ask to visit your workplace and meet up informally with your colleagues before you return to work.

Think about how you might like to share the news with your manager or your colleagues and whether you would like to tell everyone directly or have your manager or a trusted colleague tell people on your behalf. If, for example, you named your baby, you could share their name, anything you feel comfortable sharing about how they died, and anything else you feel is relevant for them to understand.

Let your employer know in advance if there is anything you would like them to do or communicate to colleagues that you feel would be helpful for you.

Being Back at Work

Getting back to work is a big decision and, once you have made it, being back at work can also be a big challenge for bereaved parents. As well as the task of settling back into your role after a period of absence during which your life changed significantly, there may be multiple other things which might feel difficult or daunting to manage at first. There might be colleagues who are still pregnant or those who visit during their own maternity leave to introduce their new baby. There might also be colleagues who have experienced the death of a baby at an earlier time. If you are the birth mother, colleagues may have seen you pregnant so might be more sensitive to your situation. For fathers, co-mothers, foster parents and adoptive parents, the loss may seem less obvious to other people and more isolating for you.

Grief can be tiring too. You may be surprised at how exhausted you feel, and you might find that you struggle to concentrate and remember things. You may find that you are very sensitive to what people say, or that you now lack confidence about making decisions. Some parents become frustrated with themselves and anxious that they can no longer cope with work. However, all of these reactions are commonplace effects of grief and should pass with time and support.

If you suddenly feel overwhelmed at work, take a break if you can. You could go for a short walk or find a quiet space to be alone. You may also find it helpful to find somewhere private to talk to a sympathetic colleague, or phone a family member, friend or the Sands helpline. If you find that being back at work is just too difficult, you could talk to your manager or employer about having some more time off or speak to your GP and see if you can take sick leave.

COPING WITH SPECIAL DATES AND ANNIVERSARIES

Certain dates and the days leading up to them may be particularly difficult to manage once you find yourself back at work; for example, the anniversary of your baby's due date or the anniversary of the day they died. Many bereaved parents feel particularly sad before or during special holidays like Christmas and Easter.

You may want to think about booking leave on those dates you expect to be especially difficult for you. This can take some of the emotional pressure off and perhaps give you an opportunity to do something different or visit a place that has special meaning for you. If these dates fall within the first 56 days after your baby's death, you could use your leave under the new Parental Bereavement (Leave and Pay) Act to do this.

Returning to work might represent a certain sense of 'normal' for you even if nothing else seems or feels normal. Falling into a routine does not mean that there won't be occasions when you need to take time off to process your ongoing grief, or that you are 'forgetting' or not honouring your baby. Returning to work is, for some parents, an important step in growing around their grief.

When you do feel ready to take this step and you are back at work, it is important to communicate both your practical and emotional needs as far as you feel able with your employer. If you are worried you might struggle to find the words without losing your composure at work, then the Sands Bereavement Support Services Team may be able to help you to explain to your employer or manager what you need.

CHAPTER 10

Breaking the Silence

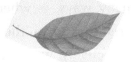

'My advice to any friends or family of someone who has experienced a stillbirth is to talk about their baby. Even years down the line. Say their name. It won't upset them because they are already thinking about them, it's just a reminder that you are too.'

Bereaved parent

'Everybody wants to talk about their baby,' says Dr Clea Harmer, CEO of Sands. She's right, and that means before, during and after birth. But for a parent whose baby dies – and for those who love and want to support them – finding the words (which is the name of just one of the recent Sands' awareness campaigns) will not come easy. It can all feel, says Clea, *just too big, too painful, too . . . no words.*

Talking helps bereaved parents stay close to the baby who

died. But if they struggle to break the thicket of silence surrounding the loss then it's no wonder that everyone else does too, even health professionals who, having been present through the trauma of the birth and death, will admit privately the thing they are most terrified of is 'saying the wrong thing'.

Because so much of the pain and trauma surrounding the death of a baby remains hidden and shrouded in an unspoken pact of silence, the whole subject of a baby dying continues to be a taboo and, in many ways, is where cancer – once only whispered about and referred to as 'the C word' or 'the Big C' – was 40 years ago. Collectively, we've smashed that taboo and it will only be collectively that we will smash this one too.

It took Pete Byrom, a bereaved dad and Sands Befriender, 14 years to 'find the right words' and talk about the death of his baby son Thomas in 2004. Now active with the Bristol-based Sands support group, Pete said it was a Facebook post by another bereaved dad who had taken part in an awareness-raising 10k charity run and who was talking, in that post, about what it felt like to be among others who knew, without words, the pain of a baby dying that smashed down his own wall of silence. He went along to a Sands support meeting and the rest, as they say, is history.

Here is Pete's story, in his own words.

THOMAS BYROM: BORN 5 JANUARY 2004

My wife, Denise, fell pregnant with our first baby in the summer of 2003. At the time we shared a house with her parents so there was a lot of excitement in the house and with my family too. We'd been trying to conceive for nearly three years and were beginning to think having children wouldn't happen for us.

Everything was going well until the thirteenth week of the pregnancy when, early on the morning of 23 September, my father-in-law burst into our bedroom to tell us that my mother-in-law had sadly passed away suddenly that morning next to him in bed. We were all devastated and for the next few weeks tried to come to terms with it while looking after my father-in-law as much as possible.

By early November things had settled down but Denise was struggling to shift what the doctors had thought was a chest infection. As it was November and the weather was cold and damp, and since Denise suffers with asthma, it was put down to a combination of everything. A couple of weeks later (when Denise was 21 weeks pregnant) I got up for work one morning to find that she'd gone and slept on the sofa as, every time she lay down, she was struggling to breathe. That, coupled with how swollen her ankles were, made me ring the GP and ask them to come out and see her. Thinking it'd be nothing serious I went to work (I worked less than a mile from home) and waited for her call to tell me what was up.

A little later that morning Denise rang me to say the doctor thought she had heart failure and had rung for a non-emergency ambulance to take her to hospital. Denise was in intensive care and at that time the doctors weren't sure she'd make it through the night.

Ironically, through all this panic, the baby was absolutely fine. The baby was scanned regularly in the first 48 hours in hospital and, from what the doctors said, seemed quite relaxed about it all! Once the doctors had drained the fluid from Denise's lungs, they began deciding what the best course of treatment was. They all agreed (renal and maternity) to put a central line into Denise's neck and put her on haemodialysis six days a week with the aim of keeping her and the baby safe for as long as possible, hoping to get through to 32 weeks when they'd then deliver the baby.

So, we set in for what we expected to be 11 weeks of this. After a couple of weeks Denise begged the doctors to release her from hospital. She wasn't getting any real rest there and we could go home and make daily trips to the hospital instead. In early December, the doctors agreed to our plan and we started our new routine.

As Christmas was approaching, I agreed one exception to Denise putting her feet up 24/7 which would be a single Christmas shopping trip. We made it through Christmas and had as quiet a time as possible, looking ahead to at least another six weeks of this same routine.

On the morning of 2 January 2004, we went to hospital for dialysis and, while Denise was having an 'oil change' (as we'd taken to calling it), I went and picked my mum up. The plan was that after the oil change, we were going over to maternity for a scan (my mum would get to see her first grandchild for the first time) and then we were going out for lunch and to buy some baby stuff. We expected, at any time, for the doctors to tell Denise she had to stay in hospital for good so wanted to do this while she still could.

The oil change was done, and we were sat in the scanning room in maternity waiting for the scan. The midwife came in and started the scan. After a minute or two we knew that she'd not found a heartbeat. The midwife said she was struggling to find one so would get a doctor to help. Everything got very tense. The doctor came in and tried but after a short time turned to us and said: 'There is no heartbeat, your baby is dead.'

Everything stopped. The room started going black and we started crying. This shouldn't have happened, I thought. We'd gotten over the worst of everything. Why is this happening to us after what we've been through?

We were taken to a side room while the midwife made arrangements for Denise to be admitted and induced that day (it was a Friday). Denise, however, refused saying she needed to tell her dad, and this wasn't something she wanted to tell him over the phone. It was arranged for us to return on Monday and for Denise to be induced then. We dropped my mum off at her house and I tried to tell my dad what had happened. Somehow I managed to drive, in a blur, back home. Denise told her dad and then the weekend just dragged on.

On Monday we returned to hospital for Denise to be induced. At just after nine o'clock on the night of 5 January, Denise gave birth to our son, Thomas. We'd both tried to stay strong for each other but when the midwife took Thomas away to clean him up and bring him back to us, we held each other and started crying. We spent some time holding Thomas in a tiny Moses basket before handing him back and moving down to the hospital's bereavement suite to begin recovery.

The next day the hospital kindly arranged a naming

185

ceremony for Thomas. We sat either side of him and held hands under the basket. We both cried throughout the short service. Just over two weeks later we had a funeral for Thomas, who is buried along with Denise's mum – she looks after Thomas as it wasn't our time to.

What helped through all this? I think the fact that our relationship was already so strong and just got stronger. We could be there for each other and to counsel family and friends through it.

What didn't help? Two things. The first was not being given any advice at the hospital and after his death about what we could and couldn't do (take pictures, dress Thomas ourselves, speak at the funeral, etc.). We were trying to do things we thought were 'allowed' rather than what we wanted. The second thing that didn't help – at all – happened a couple of days after we came home, when a midwife came out to see Denise and, as she left (knowing what we'd gone through), said: '. . . well, you are young, you can try again for another baby'.

'Another baby', says Pete, and all those who have been bereaved by the death of a much wanted baby, is never a cure for that earlier loss. It helps, of course, to become parents finally if the baby who died was your firstborn and so ameliorates the anguish of the experience in that way, but a new baby does not replace the baby who died or lessen the pain of that loss. Only growing around grief can do that.

As it happens, Pete and Denise did go on to have another baby, their son, Harrison, who is now a teenager. On the day he started school, Pete remembers walking him through the school playground and thinking to himself, 'We should be taking two to school now. He should be here with his older brother.'

He also says, during all those years when he stayed silent, not knowing how to talk about Thomas outside his immediate family, he can count on one hand the number of times anyone asked how he was doing and admits even if someone did: 'There was no time I answered that question genuinely.'

Society, bereaved parents and anyone who has been affected by the death of a baby all need to collectively break the silence not only for their own healing and sense of identity, but also to help stop babies dying unnecessarily.

Sophie Alagna (whose song, 'I Can Love You From Here', inspired the title of this book) is adamant that breaking the silence around stillbirth is not just an important part of the grieving process for bereaved parents but also crucial to saving the lives of babies who should not have died, and she has been speaking out – and breaking that taboo – since the death of her firstborn baby nine years ago.

Sophie, who tells the story of her daughter Liberty's death on page 10 and explores the legacy of that loss now a decade on, says: 'I feel very clear that if stillbirth was talked about generally, then Liberty would still be here.

'One of the first things I thought when I was told my baby had died was, *I don't understand. What is this? I'm not having a miscarriage.* There's so much focus on early miscarriage and the idea that when you get to 12 weeks, you're fine, that when I was told at nine months my baby had died, I just couldn't understand what had happened.

'I thought this was something that happened in Victorian times and so I had gone through my pregnancy with absolutely no concept this was a possibility. I'd gone through all the normal steps of a pregnancy and had all those conversations and tests, but nobody had told me that there was a potential risk of stillbirth.

'I had been concerned towards the end of the pregnancy that my baby wasn't big enough and wasn't growing and had actually gone to see health professionals and flagged that with them. So, what I feel now is that if I had had more information at that time, it could have saved my baby's life.

'I think there's an element of pregnant women being protected, even patronised, and not being trusted to hold information so there is a degree of withholding information about this risk and an idea that women can't handle it. I think it's very important that people know this is a risk so that they can look out for themselves and, maybe, more vociferously demand a scan if they have a concern.'

Sophie accepts that with the passage of all those years since Liberty died, society is starting to break taboos and shatter the secrets around those subjects which are seen as very upsetting or difficult to deal with, and agrees this is a good thing because the oppressive silence surrounding the death of a baby makes it all the more difficult to navigate the grief, the mourning and the loss.

Bereaved parents will and do contribute to the silence by censoring themselves so as not to upset other people. We all do this so that others won't feel awkward, uncomfortable or upset. But why, asks Sophie, should it be the responsibility of the parents, who have already entered into a sense of unreality following the death of their baby, to protect others from the shock and horror of the fact that babies can die too?

'It is hard to cope with any death but so much harder to cope with the death of a baby for a myriad of reasons, and the silence is one of them,' she says. 'We talk about entering a different reality, going into a different universe, entering a "secret club", which is just ridiculous, and I have to say if I am going to join any club, it's not going to be a secret for long.'

Sophie was initially shocked by people's reactions to her breaking the silence when she did speak out and says she had a feeling that, somehow, she did not conform to society's idea of what the mother of a stillborn baby would look like.

'I was supposed to look broken,' she says. 'I would turn up for work events and see people looking me up and down. I'm not sure why but my perception was that I was expected to shuffle in crying and looking mumsy in an old cardigan or, even better, disappear and not bother with the outside world again.

'You're not expected to look confident or successful. I think we're expected to shy away from society and not bother anyone with our grief again but that's not good enough for me, or indeed anybody else. It's not good enough that people whose baby has died are expected to give up on their life or their future happiness.

'I think that having a healthy relationship with death is good for everyone and that it's a good thing sometimes to confront people with reality. I think we're particularly bad at dealing with death in the UK. In the early days, I used to travel to America a lot for work and I always felt better about telling strangers there that my daughter had died than I ever did in the UK but, the truth is, being Liberty's mother is probably the biggest part of my identity and my love for her is bigger than my fear of upsetting strangers. And that's why I do speak out.'

Wider social networks can be problematic, particularly as often stillbirth is a loss unacknowledged and invalidated by society.

From 'The unique experiences of women and their families after the death of a baby', Social Work in Health Care, 2010

A Sacred Space

When a baby dies, the shock and the grief turn the natural order of things on its head. It's not natural, it's not just and it's not easy to come to terms with, however closely or distantly you are connected to and care about that loss. But there is something important others can do – they can dig deep and grow themselves by finding a way to truly empathise with grieving parents.

Sophie and Pete both talk about the importance of breaking the silence surrounding the death of a baby, not only because it makes the already daunting task of navigating through that grief less difficult than it needs to be, but also because banishing bereaved parents to some 'secret club' that nobody wants to be a member of does nothing to help them, or others affected by the death, to grieve in a healthy way. But how do we make the space for these parents to speak out and find the resilience to listen to their experiences and what they have to say?

American author and researcher Brené Brown, a research

professor at the University of Houston and the author of five *New York Times* bestsellers, who has spent over two decades studying empathy, courage, vulnerability and shame, understands that you won't know how to be around someone whose baby has died (or anyone else who is in pain) until you understand that empathy and sympathy are not the same thing, and says that to be empathic you have to make yourself vulnerable and connect with your own pain.

In a short and charming YouTube animation – which should be compulsory viewing once a day for us all ('Brené Brown on Empathy') – she highlights the important and screaming difference between empathy and sympathy: 'Empathy fuels connection, whilst sympathy drives disconnection.'

Brené recognises the hinterland that the death of a baby will catapult the people bereaved by that death to, and describes it in her animation as a deep dark hole from where those in that terrible pain are shouting from the bottom, saying: 'I'm stuck. It's dark. I am feeling overwhelmed.'

'I think of this hole as a sacred space,' she says. She's right, but you only have to move two letters around to see it is also a 'scared' space for those who find themselves in it and those who will need to join them there in order to truly empathise.

The sympathetic, imagining they are doing their best, will look over into that hole and say something crass and unintentionally cruel which almost always starts, according to Brené, with the words, 'At least . . .'

'At least you know you can get pregnant'; 'at least you can try again'; 'at least you didn't have a sick child or, worse, well, if there was something wrong with the baby . . .'

The empathic already know words won't take away the pain. And, according to Brené, instead of craning their necks to look down into the hole while keeping at a safe distance, they will climb right on down, connect with their own pain about something in their own life that landed them in that black hole, and make a real connection just by being present.

'Empathy is about feeling people. Someone who is empathic will climb down into that black hole and say, "I know what it's like down here and you're not alone."

'The truth is, rarely can a response make something better,' Brené adds. 'What makes something better is a connection. Empathy is a choice and it's a vulnerable choice. In order to connect with you I have to connect with something in me that knows that feeling.'

It is hard to see someone you love, or even a stranger, in excruciating emotional pain. It is hard to know what to say, or even whether to say anything. You'll wrack your brains trying to find the words to fix them and find a silver lining when the truth is you can't fix them, you cannot make anything better, you cannot make their pain go away and there are no silver linings. Not this time.

What you can do is allow the person who is in pain to speak, if they want to. And, says Brené, when they do just say: 'I don't know what to say right now.'

You can't fake empathy in the way you can fake sympathy. Remember how I didn't want all those flowers that were sent, in kindness and love to me, when my first baby died? I just wanted another person to say, 'I've been here. In the hinterland or the deep dark hole. And I'm here with you now.'

So, if you want to know how to be around a bereaved parent

then you either connect to something painful inside you and sit with it, just as the person in pain now is sitting with theirs, or get out of the room and don't make a painful situation any more painful.

It really is that simple. Let the person who is in pain talk about it, if they want and need to. Find the courage to do that. Acknowledge someone died. You would do so with any other bereavement.

If you do nothing else just say: 'I am sorry [insert baby's name here if you know it, and if not, just say "your baby"] died.' It is the single most powerful, most empathic, most compassionate and most meaningful thing you can say.

But if you really want to empathise with how a parent feels when their baby dies then I believe this story sums up what we all feel about it – even if we can't express it adequately. In earlier times, stillborn babies and unbaptised infants who died were not permitted burial in consecrated grounds. The story I was told, second-hand, was that of an archaeological dig in the grounds of a church somewhere in the English countryside where, on reaching the outskirts of the graveyard plot, the archaeologists were astonished to find hundreds of tiny unmarked infant inhumations.

These were the graves of the babies who had not held on to life but whose parents could not bear their exclusion from sacred ground.

The archaeologists concluded their grief-stricken parents must have snuck into the churchyard in the dead of night to give their baby what they truly deserved – the same respect, dignity and acknowledgement of the preciousness of a life, even one not lived, that we all would hope for.

FIVE THINGS YOU CAN DO TO HELP

1 Acknowledge the baby died, however long ago it happened, and say the words, 'I'm so sorry your baby died.' Say the baby's name if you know it; if you don't then ask the baby's name.

2 If you are family or a close friend, send a birthday card on the anniversary of the baby's birth.

3 Include the dead baby in the number of children a couple has had if you are talking about that.

4 If there are already children in the family, help newly bereaved parents by offering to take on some of the everyday routine responsibilities; even if it's just walking the dog or cooking a family supper for the freezer.

5 Listen. Listen. Listen.

One of the themes bereaved parents touch on, time and again, is that, often, the nurturing support they need when their baby has died doesn't come from those people they would have expected to support them, but from others they would not have imagined would be so supportive. And sometimes those others can be complete strangers.

When I told my friend, Matt, I was writing this book with Sands, he shared the following story with me which I've thought about a lot since reading it, and wondered how many other chance encounters like this one have opened the door to a painful revelation of a baby who died before, during or after birth.

This is what Matt told me: 'We got our last cat from a lovely couple who lived near Southampton. They stayed for ages when they dropped the cat off to us. It was like family visiting. Towards the end, the lady told us how she went full-term with her baby and it was a stillbirth. Apparently, a day earlier and the baby would have been fine. She was still very emotional. It was very moving, and I think the sharing of these things will help so many people, Susan.'

Matt went on to explain that the woman's first marriage had not survived the trauma and grief of the loss of their baby.

'The relationship with the first husband didn't make it. She now has a grown-up daughter with her second husband who they are clearly very proud of. She started telling us because the date of the birth of her first child was at the same time of the year that we took delivery of the cat. She said she will never forget. It was very emotional.'

It's clear to me from what Matt shared about this encounter with a stranger who, by the end of her visit, felt like a family member, that Matt and his family showed the empathy and compassion towards her story that would have made her feel her loss, all those years ago, was acknowledged and validated by this chance encounter.

In the end, that's all bereaved parents are asking for. Validation of their loss and an acknowledgement that their baby still matters.

CHAPTER 11

Memories, Rituals, Reflection and Anniversaries

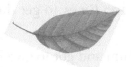

'Grief is the other side of Love; the two walk together. Understanding that is probably the single most powerful thing that helped me make peace with my grief and with my babies dying but, in all honesty, this understanding took me years . . .'

Bereaved mum

Creating memories is an important part of building the enduring bond with your baby that will allow you to grieve your loss in a healthy way and find a new normal without feeling you have betrayed the love you have for the baby you did not bring home.

All hospitals now will offer parents who lose a baby through a later miscarriage, stillbirth or neonatal death the chance to spend time with their child and create a bond by caring for them and taking photos and hand- and footprints. These first stages of memory-making can be important both at the time of death and even years later, and so while you may feel a bit awkward about creating these memories, if you have the chance then do it.

'Memories are so important as they become all we have of our babies,' says Kym, who tells the story of the death of her firstborn baby, Alfie, on page 24. 'We were fortunate; we got to spend some time with Alfie and got his hand- and footprints (if you have to do them 100 times to get them perfect, do it; trust me, it's worth it!).

'We read stories to him and got to give him a bath and get him dressed into his final outfit (some Paddington Bear pyjamas). This allowed us to feel like his parents and parent him in the only way we could at that time. This was and still is all invaluable.

'Staff also took lots of photos and videos which again are now invaluable. Even the smallest thing that may seem meaningless will be huge for parents. I know parents who have kept tissues or scraps of cotton wool they had used to gently clean their baby's skin.'

Don't feel badly if you did not start your memory-making at the hospital, either because you were too upset to or didn't know what you could or couldn't do to bond with your child. It is never too late to start making memories – including a memory box (see below) and, remember, there are no rights or wrongs. What you decide to include as a special memento need only have meaning to you, the parents.

Some families openly share their memory boxes and photos. Some prefer to keep these private. One mum told me she had recently moved a photo she had of her firstborn daughter who had died off of the mantelpiece where it was very publicly on view and over to a more discreet corner of her desk in her study. It wasn't that her dead daughter had, with the passing of the years and the subsequent birth of more children, become less important – it was more that the relationship had come to feel deeper, more enduring and more special, and not something to be passed around with the peanuts.

A lot of bereaved mums who are now many years down the road of healthy grieving will recognise this need to take back something precious and protect its importance, but, again, the only right thing to do is the thing that feels right for you.

Creating a Memory Box

Somewhere, tucked discreetly but safely in a chest of drawers or at the back of the top shelf of a wardrobe, many bereaved parents do have some kind of treasured memory box containing the precious physical evidence their baby was born and died: photos, clothing, even, as Kym describes above, the fading cotton wool balls parents have used to lovingly wash their child as they said their last goodbye.

Memories made after that hospital goodbye are, in effect, memories overlaid onto that experience of a baby dying, but that does not make them any less important. If you brought a memory box home from hospital then you have already safe-guarded important photos and documents, and you can easily add to these by including other things that keep that sense of a real baby who died alive for you. If you have a funeral for your baby, you might want to add the order of service to your memory box; if someone sent a particularly touching email, print it out and include it, the same if someone wrote or sent a moving poem. You might also want to include a lock of your baby's hair, or a card from an existing sibling. You will know what touches your heart, reminds you of the enduring bond you have with your baby and what you want to include, so trust your own feelings about this.

The Sands memory box, which is now available (at no charge) for bereaved parents in all hospitals, contains a hand-knitted blanket, two teddy bears, an *Always Loved Never Forgotten* card, support leaflets, a kit to take imprints of the baby's hands and feet and other keepsakes.

Bereaved mum, Erica Stewart, who tells the story of the death of her baby, Shane, in Chapter 5, explains the importance of having something tangible, like a memory box, to connect to your dead baby over the passing years and also the importance of deeply private rituals that, while connecting you to painful feelings, also connect you to the love you have for the child who is not with you.

'The bottom line is, nothing can bring your baby back. When Baby Shane died, it was my first experience of a major bereavement. We brought him home for a few days and had to put him into his coffin and, when we did that, I felt this stillness and thought, this is final; this is irreversible.

'Ultimately, all parents want is their baby back. It's like a kick in the teeth because you can do nothing about it; nothing is going to change this. It's irreversible. It's final. But what did help me was being able to look into his memory box whenever I wanted to; it helped me grieve and realise this was real.

'Having something tangible – like a memory box – that represents your baby is important and perhaps also doing symbolic things like lighting a candle on their anniversary or making a birthday cake or just doing whatever feels right for you.'

Having a memory box also means you have things you might want to show and share with others; including existing or subsequent children, extended family and close friends. Having something to show can also be a very good way of opening up conversations about your baby once you are ready to have them.

Looking back over the 30-plus years since Baby Shane died, Erica says her grief simply found a place to settle. Not only is it still there, she doesn't want it to go because it is that grief that connects her with Baby Shane but also with how important he is in her life. Grief is the other side of love. The two walk together.

As Erica says: 'I wouldn't have it any other way!'

LITTLE SNOWDROP

The world may never notice
If a Snowdrop doesn't bloom
Or even pause to wonder
If the petals fall too soon

(Author unknown)

A Shared Remembrance

From memorial services to flower drops, and cake bakes to the public lighting up of iconic civic buildings in blue and pink as part of the annual Baby Loss Awareness Week, many bereaved parents take great comfort from shared remembrance events which, as well as raising funds for charity or simply raising awareness of baby loss, also acknowledge their personal loss and remember their baby. Family, friends and wider work and social networks can also show support by joining parents at these events and by standing alongside them, when invited, to bear witness to whatever way they are choosing to remember their baby. And if you are also grieving for the loss of this child, sharing in these remembrance activities can help you to acknowledge and show your own sadness.

Nationwide in the UK, there are many bereavement support memorial events run by Sands – including the Sands Garden Event and Lights of Love. Both events are for bereaved parents and families to remember their baby and celebrate their life. The first Sands Garden Event was launched in 2000 and takes place at the National Memorial Arboretum in Staffordshire.

Winter remembrance events are also held. The first Lights of Love service took place in 2004 at St Paul's Church in Knightsbridge where the Christmas tree was decorated with cards bearing messages dedicated to babies and loved ones who have died. Since then, more secular and diverse events have been held around the UK in memorial gardens and outside spaces, such as petal drops in rivers, tree planting, fields of windmills and lantern walks.

A great deal of thought is given to the format of events, so that they allow parents and families a chance to reflect and remember, including a quiet time to reflect on your own loss and grief, before moving on to those elements that allow you to celebrate your enduring bond with your child.

Even the Sands' annual conference poignantly makes space for a time of reflection; at the 2019 conference bereaved parents were given tiny flowers attached to blank card where they could write the name of their baby or babies. The sorrow in the room, quiet by this stage, was palpable as parents queued to gently place their memorial flowers on a length of green carpet representing a garden. At the end of the ritual, the sight of all those tiny flowers and names was a poignant one. For more information on the annual events run by Sands, please see the website: www.sands.org.uk

The way you want to acknowledge your baby and their ongoing meaning in your life will be a personal choice and one you may want to keep private or share with others so they can join you in those acknowledgments and celebrations. Maybe you have a picnic on the baby's birthday and invite the whole family, or perhaps you organise a fundraising event in your baby's name.

There is no right or wrong here. Do what feels right for you. I lost three babies and most evenings I light a group of three candles. I would be lighting these candles anyway at the end of a busy day but, for me, there is something symbolic and meaningful in that grouping of three that reminds me of a bond that is enduring, albeit private.

If, one year, you try a new way of celebrating your enduring bond, but it doesn't feel quite right, don't worry. Just do something different the next time you want to acknowledge a birthday or the fact the family is still missing and will always miss someone.

Family occasions like birthdays, anniversaries and holidays, and all the events and social gatherings that punctuate the year, can feel very painful, especially in those first years after coming home from hospital without your baby. You can counter these feelings of sadness by arranging a dedicated celebration of the baby and share that moment with your partner, with friends or your wider social circle if that feels right for you.

A LASTING TRIBUTE

With all the digital tools now at our disposal it has never been easier to create a lasting tribute to your baby, which will be a reflection of the enduring bond you have created. A Sands Always Loved tribute, for example, is a wonderful and lasting way to remember your baby. In partnership with the memorial website charity MuchLoved, we can provide you with a way of creating a tribute website which, if you wish, can also be used to raise funds for Sands.

An Always Loved tribute is an entirely safe space to help you remember and reflect, making it part of the 'loving you from here' journey. You can easily add and display a whole range of information and memorabilia, including stories, messages of condolence, pictures, music and video clips. You can also write an online journal. Your free online memorial dedicated to your precious baby can be shared with family and friends or kept completely private if you'd prefer. The choice, as always, is yours and, again as always, there is no right or wrong. The only right is what feels right for you. Find out more at: www.sands.org.uk/always-loved-tributes

An Enduring Bond

British actor, David Haig, and his wife, Julia Gray, were already busy parents to four children, Alice then 11, Caroline, 8, Fred, 5 and Harry, 2, when their fifth child, Grace, was stillborn in 1996 – on David's fortieth birthday.

David, a Sands Ambassador, and Julia, a former actress and now a trained counsellor working with young people, have worked tirelessly and for over two decades to support other bereaved parents so, as a couple, they are more than qualified to explore the idea of an enduring bond (or 'loving you from here') through the long lens of the passage of time.

Here are their thoughts, shared during a joint interview, about their experience, about the impact of time passing and about the huge contribution Grace has made to their entire family's lives.

GRACE: BORN 20 SEPTEMBER 1996

'It was a terrible shock although I had had a sense that something wasn't right for about a week before Grace was born at 39 weeks plus 3 days,' says Julia. 'I was at home when I had a visit from the midwife and said, "I think you had better check this baby is still alive."'

Julia, who had given birth to their first daughter, Alice, in hospital but then had three successful home births before Grace, adds: 'I was completely innocent of anything that could remotely go wrong. We'd had four relatively straight-forward pregnancies, so it just didn't occur to me for a minute and I had never ever read anything about stillbirths.

'So, then I thought well, what happens now? I had this weird feeling that if the baby had died, it would be assimilated back into me. I don't know what I thought, but I went with the midwife to hospital and David followed a bit later. We stayed at the hospital overnight. It was the worst night of my life. It was desolate.

'I kept looking at myself in the mirror in the bathroom thinking I just want this over; I want it out. I just wanted them to knock me out and give me a caesarean. I didn't want to feel anything.

'Now, I can't remember anything about the birth, except the last five minutes. We were looked after so badly I can't even begin to describe it. They were just so callous and insensitive.'

The midwife who had taken Julia in had told the staff to let her know as soon as she went into labour, but nobody did, which meant David had to run frantically down the corridors to find someone and that the midwife, who had been doing a clinic elsewhere, arrived after the birth.

'After Grace was born, I didn't really want to see her but I must have read something somewhere about the importance of looking at and holding the baby so I did and then, of course, I couldn't stop.

'There was something extraordinary about how instinctively you get a map in your mind's eye about every single feature, which was something I needed to imprint. Once I had done that she was put into a cot. I didn't know then I could have done other things; I didn't think about the children coming in to see her or that I could bath her. I hadn't taken any clothes in, so she was wrapped in a hospital towel and those are the pictures that I have of her.

'After about three hours, I thought I think I can say goodbye now.'

David and Julia did have another baby, another baby girl who they named Connie. 'I didn't want my fertile years to end on such a sad note,' Julia explains.

'One of the things that has always interested me about grief of any sort is its potential complexity in relationship to the people suffering the grief,' says David. 'I always remember when my sister died, aged 22, my mother leaving the cemetery hand-in-hand with my sister's boyfriend and my father walking behind, rejected.

'Death can disunite, rather than unite. It didn't disunite me and Julia, but it was certainly complex. My experience of Grace's death was subtly different and complicated. I think because my sister had died young, I was less shocked that Grace had died than Julia was.

'Nothing shocks me. When people die of cancer or die in stillbirth, no death shocks me. The absolute random lottery of life and fate and chance after my sister's death made me feel not that it was inevitable but that it wasn't a surprise. Of course, emotionally, Grace's death was appalling but it wasn't, for me, shocking.

'The other difference is the experience in the hospital. I just remember the colour grey as a dominating metaphor and the desolate view across London from the window of the room on the fourteenth floor where Julia was giving birth; the paper-thin walls, through which we could hear the celebrations of a successful birth, and running down the corridor, trying to alert anybody to the fact that Julia was actually giving birth to death and that there was no one there to help her.

'So, again from the father's point of view, and this is about the father being on the outside, I was witnessing something that should never have happened, was appallingly mismanaged and devastating emotionally for the person I loved.

'When Grace was born – apart from recognising the inevitable genetic influence of my mother whose chin and wide cheeks is apparent in all our children – her face was grey, shading to white. The skin was going cold and when you touched it, your finger would stick to it and then, as you pulled your finger away, the skin goes with it.

'I was acutely aware of this being a dead human being and, as a result, did not want to carry her which was profoundly different from Julia's response. I looked, and I touched, and I hated mortality and the fateful lottery of shitting on human beings in this situation, which is so unjust and so erratic, and so unpredictable.

'After the baby went, my memories are much hazier until the funeral and seeing the clear whiteness of the box and the tiny size of it.'

Grace's funeral was an intimate one with just David and Julia and the vicar present. The couple's existing children did not attend, and Julia also told her sisters not to come, although she says now she had sort of wished they would have just turned up in spite of her saying don't, and that maybe telling them not to was really about protecting their feelings.

'It is a regret of mine now that the children did not come to the funeral but, at the time, it felt like it was a very private thing between me and David,' Julia explains. 'But with hindsight, I wish they had been there. It's quite difficult for a child to grasp what has happened when all they saw was my pregnant stomach and then me being upset for a long time.'

David says, unlike Julia, he does not regret the children not attending. 'We're a family who talk about virtually everything, so the fact that neither of us embraced the children coming as a possibility means we must have made an instinctive choice about that,' he says.

'My feeling about long-term grief is not to try to get over it. You always carry it in parallel to your life and you get used to sharing your life with that awareness, otherwise there is a temptation to suppress, which can never be healthy.

'The cruelty of time passing is that I miss my sister and Grace less than I used to because time has done what is its kindest and cruellest thing which is that time both anaesthetises and distances but, at the same time, it helps people survive.

'If it wasn't for time, we'd all be gnashing our teeth and wailing in the biblical sense over the losses we experience through life until we die, which would make life impossible. So, it's a balance between getting used to the loss and not missing the person as much as you used to and forgiving time for doing that.

'But as I miss my sister, Karen, and Grace and my father, and all the other people in my life who have died, slightly less as time goes by, then symbolic memorials become more important.

'We've just built a big Japanese garden at the bottom of the garden which is called "Grace's Garden 2" and all the family use it. It's a very cool place; we've got electricity, and we all go and watch television and talk down there and it's very beautiful.

'We had built a tiny, first garden for Grace immediately after her death and in the pictures of us all standing there, we all have very solemn faces. If you saw the faces of the people enjoying her new garden now, they are animated and joyful because time has forgiven, in a sense, the agony most of the time – not all of the time because sometimes it will suddenly hit you – then it allows us to derive pleasure and joy from the second memorial.'

David and Julia have a line from a Van Morrison song called 'In the Garden', which they have included in both of Grace's memorial gardens which, they say, unite the gardens across the passage of time: 'You and I and nature, in the garden, wet with rain.'

Following our conversation for this book, Julia sent me a short message which I think sums up why the enduring bond bereaved parents work so hard to create and maintain for the babies they don't bring home is such an important part of coming to terms, as David has described, in a healthy way with their grief: 'We were just saying how much we value the opportunity to focus on Grace and the massive contribution she has made to our lives and our family, in her absence.'

Creating an enduring bond with the baby, or, for some, babies, who died is a choice. It is not going to happen by chance or even with the passing of time. You need to decide this is something you want; namely a deep and meaningful and ongoing relationship with someone who is not here and who did not leave any trace of their personality, so you are also going to need to imagine how they would have grown up and who they would have become.

They say that practice makes perfect, and that holds true for creating an enduring bond. Even if it feels strange at first, do something that makes you think of your baby and, the following day, do it again. Joanna, who talked about the death of her twin boys on page 123 says, 'When we sign cards, we both put two little stars. It's just a very gentle way of keeping our children alive; talking about them by name, not being scared to talk about them and not just on anniversaries.'

I light my three candles and like to wear three rings on my right hand. Another family may pick a random day – not the anniversary of a birth or a death but a day for celebration – and gather for an annual picnic or walk on the beach to talk about and remember the missing member of the family group.

It can feel strange, at first, to create these rituals and remembrances and symbolic habits, but they are what underpin the enduring bond and encourage it to flourish and, at some point, once they have become woven into the fabric of your everyday life, then just like David and Julia above, you won't ever have to question your enduring bond, no matter what has happened to you since or how many years have gone by. It will have become just a fact of your life.

CHAPTER 12

Thinking About Trying Again?

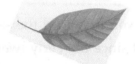

"Hope" is the thing with feathers
That perches in the soul
And sings the tune without the words
And never – stops at all

'"Hope" is the Thing with Feathers', Emily Dickinson

When a baby dies before, during or after birth, pregnancy for bereaved parents will never again be a time of any kind of joyful innocence. My admiration for the courage of those who do try again is enormous and, of all the stories bereaved parents who have gone on to a successful birth – and to bring their baby home from hospital – have shared with me, the one I first heard when writing an article for the Press Association long before this book was commissioned is the following one, which left me in awe of this family, but especially mum, Jayne.

I was asked to interview Jayne over the phone and because she now has a young family – two boys – we agreed to do it on a Friday evening while her husband, Steven, did bath time and put the boys to bed. We started our conversation at around 6pm and concluded it close to 11pm after taking a couple of breaks for Jayne to kiss her boys goodnight and for me to change the batteries in my tape recorder and find a new notebook.

Twice, through the incredible story of her determination to become a mum, I found myself close to tears. And when you read her story below, you may find the same happens to you. I have been a journalist since my early twenties, almost 40 years, and must have spoken to and interviewed thousands of people, often telling harrowing stories, over those years. But Jayne's honesty, eloquence and openness in reliving, in minute detail, the decade-long challenge to start her family and become a mum comes into my mind frequently. I had never heard such an inspiring story of determination and resolve.

JAYNE'S STORY

Passengers boarding the easyJet flight EZY8704 from Tenerife to Gatwick were alarmed to see, as they boarded the plane, a couple in the front row seats holding hands and sobbing. The young woman, clearly pregnant and struggling to keep her distress under control, had her head hidden in her hands.

'Is she all right? Is she scared of flying?' the older woman boarding in the seat behind the crying mother-to-be asked as she pushed her cabin bag into the overhead locker.

The husband, ashen and wild-eyed with disbelief, shock and the couple's shared grief, simply shook his head.

Not all the boarding passengers were as sympathetic. One man tutted and muttered something about people pulling themselves together. Most just looked away.

Another pregnant woman struggled down the aisle, cradling her own baby bump protectively, which proved too much for the already sobbing woman who gave in to another wave of body-wracking grief.

What she, her husband, the cabin crew and, soon, the kindly lady behind the couple knew was that the baby girl inside her – a baby she had struggled through 10 years of miscarriages and, finally, IVF treatment to conceive and hold on to in utero to 30 weeks' gestation and the last trimester of pregnancy – was dead.

Jayne and Steven could not have been happier on their outbound flight. Their obstetrician had confirmed Jayne was safe to fly and the couple had packed their bags to take a week in the sun and enjoy a 'babymoon' holiday before the pregnancy – a pregnancy they could still scarcely believe was finally happening – moved into the excitement of the last two months.

But the couple's dream of finally having a baby was shattered when, just a few days into their holiday, Jayne realised she could no longer feel Poppy moving, and when an emergency scan at the local Spanish hospital confirmed the news no couple ever wants to hear.

'We had been so happy when we set out on that holiday,' says Jayne. 'We'd never got this far in seven previous pregnancies, all of which had ended in the first few weeks when either there was no heartbeat or the baby had died, and this was the first time, in almost 10 years, we both could believe this is our baby; this is really happening.

'I had a little baby bump that I was so proud of. I loved looking and being pregnant and, although I was too scared to have sex with my husband or do anything that might jinx our luck, just before we flew out for our babymoon, we had had a 4D scan where you can actually see a 3D image of your baby moving in real time.

'There she was, jumping about, yawning and sticking her tongue out. Everything was normal and I had never felt so happy as I felt at the airport on the day we flew out to Tenerife. I felt like the luckiest woman alive.'

Jayne's feelings of elation and sheer joy at being pregnant and a mum-to-be began to dissipate when the little voice in her head telling her something was not right started to become more insistent.

'Poppy was a very active baby and I knew she was not moving as much, if at all. I tried everything – drinking fizzy drinks and doing jumping jacks because I thought, I hoped, maybe she was just sleeping and that maybe I could jolt her awake. But in my heart, I knew something was very wrong.

'When I woke in the night to go to the toilet, I could not feel her normal kicks or any movement at all and I started to panic. I woke Steven up and he said we would go to the local hospital and get checked in the morning. By the time we were sitting waiting for the scan, the anxiety was bubbling up.

'The doctor came in with an archaic-looking monitor; none of the medical staff at the hospital had good English and we did not speak Spanish and when the scan picked up a heart-beat I knew, instantly, it wasn't the galloping heartbeat of a baby which I had heard so many times before, it was my heartbeat. The doctors could not find any other heartbeat and although I didn't want to believe it, I knew in that moment Poppy had died.'

Jayne watched and listened in disbelief as the doctor delivered the devastating news in broken English and felt time itself stop as her husband, the man who had been a rock through the rollercoaster of so many disappointments, each time they had lost a pregnancy, fell to the floor.

'Steven was a broken man. It's all a bit of a blur when I think back to that time, but I remember thinking he's doing enough crying for the both of us and I can't fall apart now. I need to get home. We walked out of that hospital completely devastated. I felt responsible, like it was all my fault and I had brought nothing but heartbreak to Steven and both our families. I was even angry that we had decided to have the IVF which had resulted in being pregnant with Poppy.'

Jayne and Steven cried together that night. They knew they needed to and should sleep but they also knew this would be the only time it would be just the three of them – Mum, Dad and Poppy – and their one and only chance to deal solely with their own grief because coming home would mean facing the grief of their families and friends.

It's difficult to hear just how hard it was for the devastated couple to get home to the UK to deliver their stillborn baby. There were no flights available which meant they had to stay on at their resort another day, and even when they finally did board the plane, after the horrors of queuing with everyone else (including pregnant women and other families), they had not, initially, been seated together.

The shock, the horror, the pain and the tragedy of an imminent stillbirth is not something society can handle as the couple's horrendous journey home shows. When they asked if they could sit together, another passenger eventually changed seats but not before several others had declined. And when they landed at Gatwick and made their way to the luggage carousel, an unexplained delay meant standing, holding on to one another and trying to hold back a public display of their grief for another unnecessary hour.

Jayne's mum, Christine, and stepdad, Jonathan, himself a doctor, were waiting in the arrivals hall; both looked white with the strain of the news and the grief about to unleash. Steven's dad, Edwin, was waiting for them to get home too.

'Mum was still hoping the Spanish doctors had got it wrong, but I knew Poppy was gone. I couldn't face going home where we'd decorated the nursery, so we went, instead, to the airport chapel. It was Mother's Day the next day and, while other families were out buying flowers and cards, we were talking about where Poppy should be buried and what kind of funeral we should have once she had been born.'

THE BIRTH

'You think you can prepare yourself for this. You think when you've had a few days to prepare, a few days knowing your baby has died and she will be born dead you will find a way to make your peace with that, but you don't; you can't,' says Jayne.

'We chose to go to the local hospital which had been so supportive to us throughout all our previous pregnancies – and losses – to have Poppy. I had been booked in there for a C-section had we gone to term so even the idea of a natural birth instead was a shock to me.

'The doctors gave me a tablet to get things started and we settled into our own little room; Steven, me and Mum. We played cards to pass the time and although, for the most part, I felt numb, I did keep thinking if there is a God, why has he put me through this? Why am I about to go through all this pain? Why does this have to be my birthing experience?'

There are no words, says Jayne, to describe what happened or how she felt next. You cannot hurry a stillbirth and so the lengthy labour churned up so many emotions; sad, beautiful, surreal and bizarre.

'Poppy had always been so active in the womb, we had nicknamed her Supergirl and when she was finally born, she came out, arm first, like Wonder Woman; I just loved that,' Jayne recalls.

'The birth itself was a relief. I had been sick everywhere and it was just such a relief all that was over. We had thought we would call our baby Isobel but when she came out and I looked at her I thought she's not an Isobel, she's a Poppy and Steven agreed.

'And finally, we knew why she had died. There was a knot in the umbilical cord. There was nothing wrong with her;

there was nothing wrong with my womb. We did not need to agree to a post-mortem. And so, as devastating as it was, we had an answer and the one thing we had to accept was that it was nobody's fault.'

Deep down and over the coming days Jayne was angry with somebody and that somebody was Poppy. 'I was angry with her for a while; angry she had been naughty – she was always turning and wiggling; and the cord had ended up knotted. If only she had stayed still. We had so much love for her and she would have had such a lovely life with us. I was cross with her. And angry she had died the way she had. I couldn't understand why we had been allowed, by God, I suppose, to get so far into the pregnancy. I thought life just sucks, and there's nothing you can do.'

Jayne says her daughter was not only perfectly formed but, with her shock of dark hair and long, slender fingers, beautiful too. 'I thought about how we would never know what colour her eyes would be or what her voice would have sounded like. I wanted to believe she had been given to us for a reason and, in the end, I told myself that since God has to take some babies back, he took Poppy because he knew Steven and I are a strong couple and we would eventually cope with that loss whereas it could tear another couple apart.'

When something as desperately sad, devastating and, as was the case with Poppy, random as the death of a much-wanted baby happens, there is no choice but to start bargaining and trading with some higher power – imagined or, if you have faith, real – because the brain cannot comprehend that something so cruel, so significant and with such lasting consequences can happen for absolutely no good reason.

Those most affected by the loss, the parents, of course, but equally close family, friends who love them, existing siblings, work colleagues and anyone whose life has been touched by the sadness, will take their lead from the parents in trying to understand what has happened, and why, and so this negotiating with the reasons why, and just as importantly the inevitable question 'Why me?' is a deep-seated reaction to the shock, the unfairness and the dread of a long-haul grieving process that can feel as if it will never end.

Like everyone who has been through a stillbirth, Jayne and Steven searched hard for the shreds of anything they could hang on to in order to survive the loss and try to take something unshakeable home with them. And for this couple, it was the funeral.

'Steven said, well, since I will never walk her down the aisle, I want to carry the coffin; at least let me do this for my daughter. We both knew there was nothing we could have done to have changed what happened or the fact Poppy was dead. We had to tell ourselves she was where she was always going to be and there was nothing either of us could do to change that.

'We had to hold on to knowing that for the short time she had been with us she had felt loved and I did feel blessed to think that she would, somehow, know that.'

TRYING AGAIN

Like all mothers who have lost a baby, Jayne left the hospital in a daze of conflicting emotions. She knew she could never replace Poppy but that desperate feeling to have her own child had only become stronger.

'We had come so far, and it had taken so many years, I knew that if we were going to try again then we would have to try straight away,' she recalls. 'We would be grieving for Poppy anyway, however long we waited, and we were both completely united in that grief and in our determination not to give up now; we could not let that – being childless – happen to us after we had been through so much and I could no longer imagine going to an adoption meeting. I just didn't know if I would feel the same towards a child who was not my own and that wouldn't be fair on any child.'

Nobody really wanted the couple to try to get pregnant again so soon; not the clinic where they had gone through IVF treatment combined with genetic screening to get pregnant with Poppy and, although they were supportive, not their families or friends.

'Everyone wanted us to wait. The clinic was shocked we wanted to try again; they told us we needed time to grieve and should wait. But I didn't need time to grieve. I knew I would always grieve for my daughter but that I would also grieve for the child I still didn't have.'

Just six weeks after Poppy's death, the couple underwent another round of IVF which failed. 'It was heartbreaking,' says Jayne. 'We had hit the jackpot the first time with Poppy and we really had to work hard to pick ourselves up from another disappointment. I felt frustrated and angry; I thought my body is a failure, I am a failure.'

Jayne says underlying the grieving for her lost daughter and the failed IVF attempt was a growing panic that Poppy would be the only baby she would ever have. So, after allowing her body to return to normal just enough to have one period, she and Steven went back to the clinic.

'Again, they told us to wait. They said we should come back in six months, even better in a year, but we were very firm and said we are not waiting. I was feeling thwarted and nobody was getting in my way,' says Jayne.

When Jayne turned up for the IVF transfer of a healthy embryo – her third IVF treatment – she carried Poppy's teddy bear with her.

'We'd had seven early miscarriages before going down the route of combined genetic screening with IVF and Poppy had shown me that I could get past the first trimester without miscarrying, so I tried to feel more confident when the pregnancy test showed the transfer had worked and I was pregnant again.

'But it was a very, very hard pregnancy. I was still grieving for Poppy and every time I had a bleed – and I had a big one at 11 weeks – I thought we were going to lose the baby. My anxiety levels were through the roof and even though I was having counselling and weekly scans, I couldn't shake the fear that something would go wrong again.

'In the end, the doctors were so concerned about my anxiety they agreed that this new baby should be delivered by C-section at 34 weeks. A close friend had just lost her baby on her due date and I couldn't go another day with the fear I would lose my baby too.

'We didn't know whether we were having a boy or a girl – we wanted to have what my mum calls "a joyful surprise" and so when my son William was born, we had that but also it was lovely, and sad – because of Poppy – all at the same time.

'Everyone in that room cried when he was delivered, even the consultant. Steven cried and I was in complete shock. I could not believe I finally had a baby. I kept expecting them to say something was wrong and so the real challenge for me then was coming to terms with having a baby that was OK.'

Jayne says the joy and the relief of having a baby were overshadowed by feeling guilty that that baby was not Poppy: 'I had a really difficult time and struggled far more than I realised I would. William was the spitting image of Poppy which was hard and having a new baby is exhausting, even when you have a good baby.

'I was full of joy and relief that I had finally done it, but it didn't stop me grieving for and feeling the loss of the baby I had lost.'

THIS HAPPY ENDING

This rollercoaster of bittersweet emotions is a challenge in itself. When a family that has lost a baby through stillbirth or neonatal death does come home with another baby, there is enormous pressure on them to come home, hang up the baby bunting, shout their joy from the rooftops and act as if the happy ending cancels the trauma and the grief that has gone before.

But that's not how feelings work and so for new mums like Jayne, coping with the enormous adjustment to a new (and much-wanted) baby and other people's expectations that she would be ecstatically happy now – while still grieving the loss of an earlier child – is a huge challenge and one she sums up in just two words: 'beautifully hard'.

When William reached the milestone of his first birthday, the couple took the plunge again and started another round of IVF treatment. And again, it worked, which meant that the following year they came back from the hospital, once again, cradling a newborn and a brother for William whom they named Oliver.

The family, says Jayne, is now complete.

The couple, who were by now in their late thirties and who had spent a decade trying to have a family, flirted with the idea of a third and final baby but decided they did not want to put themselves, their boys or their extended family through any more trauma.

For now, Jayne has stopped the bereavement counselling; life with two young sons is just too hectic she says and, besides that, she adds, she wants to be happy for her boys. But memories of Poppy, the pain of thinking about memories the now completed family will never make with her, and the sorrows of that loss are, as they are for all bereaved parents, never far from the surface. Daily. And regardless of going on to have more children.

Sands 'Pregnancy After Loss' Groups

'Psychological distress persisted into subsequent pregnancies when parents reported differing emotions (e.g. relief and worry, hopeful optimism, and panic attacks or depressive symptoms).

Women tended to report volatile emotional states, whereas fathers tended to report suppression of their feelings. Parents were afraid to prepare for the birth of their subsequent baby and avoided general antenatal classes because they felt, as parents, they were outside the boundaries of normality. Some women struggled to differentiate their dead baby's identity from their subsequently born live baby.'

From the 2018 *Lancet* series on stillbirth

Many of the 100-plus monthly support groups run by Sands volunteers and Befrienders are dedicated to the challenge of getting pregnant again and supporting parents through their understandable fear and dread that another baby will die.

On the morning I interview Scottish mum, Fiona Donald, who is the chair of the Aberdeen Sands support group and a long-time Befriender, who has made it her personal mission to educate healthcare practitioners on best practice following baby loss since the deaths of her baby daughter Gemma in 1997 and, tragically, her second daughter, Sarah, too in 1998, she tells me there is a 'Trying Again' Sands group meeting that evening which she will attend. She adds that when other bereaved parents learn she has survived the death of not one, but two babies, and then went on to have two more children, they feel encouraged, thinking: *Well, if you can survive the death of two, I can survive the death of one.*

Here, in her own words, is Fiona's story and, running through it, her key message to bereaved parents who plan to get pregnant again, which is to tell the healthcare professionals exactly what you need and make sure you get it.

GEMMA LOUISE DONALD: BORN 27 FEBRUARY 1997, DIED 24 MARCH 1997 AND SARAH JOANNE DONALD: BORN 19 MARCH 1998, DIED 30 APRIL 1998

I hadn't got a baby and all my friends had and that just drove me on. I thought I am not going to be defeated. I want a baby. I don't want a baby to replace the babies who died, I just want a baby.

I never thought it would happen the way it happened; I just thought you would go for a baby and you would get one. We had decided as a couple we would travel the world first and so when we did come to starting our family, and it went wrong, we had my age against us. I was 35 when I had Gemma, 36 when I had Sarah, 37 when I had Lauren and 40 when I had my youngest, Mitchell. And I had two miscarriages too; one early miscarriage in 1995 before Gemma and a second later one, at 16 weeks, before Mitchell.

When Gemma died, she was in the children's hospital in Birmingham where she'd fought for three-and-a-half weeks and, in a weird kind of way, when she died, we felt relieved. She'd been born, via caesarean, with a major heart defect and while we wanted her, we knew she would not have had a good quality of life.

Gemma's care was great, but after 25 days, she lost her fight.

After Gemma died, it was definitely the support of friends and family that got us through, plus I found a Sands support group. And then I got pregnant with our second daughter, Sarah, and her death was a big shock because she was here, in our arms, and then suddenly she was gone.

Sarah had picked up a virus at six weeks old which gave her myocarditis; and again, it was the support of family and friends that got us through.

Our friends definitely changed when our babies died. I made a lot of new friends through Sands who were comfortable with me talking endlessly about it. Some friends disappeared altogether but others rose to the occasion.

I remember going for a scan when I was pregnant with Lauren and the sonographer asked why there was a green sticker on my file. When I told her Gemma and Sarah had both died, she started crying and asked me, 'How do you get through that? What do you need?' I told her I didn't need anything – I had the Sands Trying Again group support.

When Lauren was born so many people came to see me; one day there were 20 people crowded into the room. They were all people who had supported me through that pregnancy.

After Sarah died, I had changed GPs and complained about the health visitor who had told me she was too busy to help me that day when I rang to say something was wrong. She was sent on extra training and I have made it a bit of a mission to help educate health professionals ever since then. I know that a different response from that health visitor would not have changed the outcome for Sarah, but it was not a good response and I put my energy into highlighting that.

For Gemma, we had a small funeral service in Aberdeen; for Sarah we had a much bigger funeral even though I hadn't wanted one. I remember walking in, seeing her coffin there and walking out again. But my dad had told me we should have a service and so I went back in.

I was part of a church group at that time which had been very supportive, but I never blamed God. I didn't think he had anything to do with it, but I just hoped he would help us get through it. To be honest, I didn't think anything; I was just so numb with the shock of it.

When I was pregnant again with Lauren, who is now 21, I was always looking for scans. I made a 'deal', if that's the right word, with the hospital to have as many scans as I needed, including echo scans to monitor the heart. I just had to phone the hospital and I could go up for a scan, so I don't think I really bothered with midwives until the last few weeks of the pregnancy. All my care throughout that preg- nancy was hospital-based. Going to Sands groups was also a big support through the pregnancy.

Once I could feel her moving at 16 weeks, I felt a lot better. And once she was born, I got her echo scanned once a month for a whole year until eventually they said to me, she's one now and she's fine, her heart is physically fine.

I tell other bereaved parents now to go along to the hospital, say what you want, and they will do it after you've had a loss. I've had Sands' parents phone me up and say, 'I'm in a lot of pain and I don't know what to do,' so I have actually phoned the ward for them and arranged for them to go to hospital to get checked and reassured that everything is fine.

We have a Next Time Sands meeting tonight and that's what we will tell the parents who come along. If you want a scan every week, get a scan every week. They're happy to do it, but you have to ask. All of us who have lost babies know you have the scan, get the reassurance, go home feeling happy and then wake up the next day thinking everything was fine yesterday, but wondering whether it is still fine today. That's one of the constant stresses of getting pregnant again after your baby has died.

After I'd had Lauren and Mitchell – and this is something we talk about at Sands meetings a lot – a lot of people think your worries are over and you're having a total restart. But that's not the case because when your baby has died, there is always an underlying anxiety about the children you have had since.

I was still walking Mitchell to school when a lot of his class-mates were allowed to walk alone. I remember him asking, 'Why won't you let me walk on my own?' He kept asking and one day I just said, 'Because I've already lost two children and I'm not losing another one.' And Lauren's 21 now and driving. It's a constant worry that your child is going to die and one that never really goes away.

If You Want to Try Again

If you do decide that having another baby is the right decision for you, it is best to wait until any medical issues have been resolved. These could include underlying conditions for the birth mother, illness during the previous pregnancy or scars from the birth. You might also want to wait until your six-week check-up before you try again. Your baby's post-mortem examination might also reveal specific problems so try to think about all these things before trying for another baby.

While people may assume that if you do find yourself pregnant again you will want to shout it from the rooftops, the truth for most bereaved parents is very different. It can feel very difficult to share the news of your new pregnancy or to allow yourself to get excited about having a baby. And, as with grief itself, you and your partner may not experience the same feelings about this new pregnancy at the same time, which can also be very challenging.

Having had a personal experience of baby loss, you now know that not all pregnancies end happily and, of course, if you have existing children, they might remember the time that their sibling died and, just like you, be very afraid that this might happen again. You might find that your child wants to revisit conversations you had when the baby died and that they now have more questions and feelings that they need to explore with you. It's important to find out what your child remembers and then try to fill in any gaps in their understanding if you can. If this feels too distressing for you, perhaps a family member or friend can help, so don't be afraid to ask.

ANTENATAL CARE

Some parents will choose to go back to the same maternity unit that cared for them when their baby died, while others do not want to relive the memories of their baby's death in the same place. If you do not have the choice to go to another hospital and find the prospect of attending the same hospital too distressing, you can ask to be under the care of a different consultant and a different team of midwives from those you had previously.

It is natural to want to be extra cautious and to feel very, very anxious throughout a subsequent pregnancy, so if there is anything at all about your new pregnancy that is worrying you, it is essential to tell a member of your healthcare team. In addition to the usual antenatal clinics, some maternity units run special clinics or drop-in sessions for bereaved parents who are expecting another baby, where they understand the anxiety and pain of a new pregnancy and can provide extra reassurance and check-ups. And, of course, there are many Trying Again groups run by Sands where other parents will know exactly how anxious you feel.

If you are the birth mother, you might feel especially anxious throughout the entire pregnancy and these feelings will be exacerbated as you reach the point in your pregnancy when your previous baby died. You can ask for extra health checks to help reassure you through this difficult time. Your notes should be marked with a special sticker or alert to indicate that you have had a baby who died.

Sands provides special stickers or alerts to health professionals to use (see Appendix, page 278). This is so that everyone involved in your care is aware that you might need extra support. If you go to antenatal classes, tell the person facilitating the class that your previous baby died. They too can then be sensitive to your needs and understand why you might have additional concerns to some of the other non-bereaved parents attending the same class.

RELATING TO THE NEW BABY

For most parents, planning a nursery and choosing clothes for a baby they are expecting is an exciting experience and one they can share not only with their partner but with their wider circles of family and friends. When your previous baby has died, it can be difficult to feel confident enough to make any preparations for the arrival of your baby. Again, it is important that you speak to someone about your anxieties. Maybe ask a family member or friend for practical help in putting together your hospital bag ready for the birth and ask someone who has supported you through the loss of your previous baby to shop for baby clothes and equipment with you when you are ready to do that. You may feel more comfortable to wait until after your baby is born before you make any extra preparations and that is fine if that is what you prefer.

It is not unusual to find that you feel afraid of loving the new baby and of forming any strong attachments until you are confident that he or she is alive and well and will be coming home from the hospital with you. It is totally natural to have these fears. And you might also find that you are extremely protective of the new baby when they are born (see below).

Think carefully with your partner and your healthcare team about what you would like from your birth plan and make sure you let those caring for you know what you need. When the anxious feelings start to feel overwhelming, talk to your Sands supporters, therapist or healthcare team about your fears so they can reassure you and, remember, everyone taking care of you and your baby now just wants you to come home from hospital this time with your healthy baby.

233

ANXIOUS PARENTING

That constant anxiety through any subsequent pregnancy that Fiona talks about, as her story shows, does not depart with the happiness of bringing a baby born after baby loss back home. In fact, it never goes away. But having a baby who does come home from hospital with you does, according to researchers, lower the risk of life-long depression following a baby's death.

One study found that the single most significant factor influencing symptoms of depression following a baby's death was not having another baby within three years of that loss. They also noted that this risk of serious depression increased again when the stillborn baby was the third and yet again if it was the fourth child born into the family, presumably because at this point and in contrast to when the baby who died was the first-born, hope for a subsequent and successful pregnancy is diminished by the ticking of the biological clock and the feeling that time is no longer on your side.

And while research exploring whether children born into a family after the death of a baby are at risk of 'over smothering' by overprotective parents is inconclusive – a concept some academics refer to as the 'vulnerable child' or the 'replacement child' – there is not a single mother who has contributed to this book who does not admit it was very hard to allow their child the usual freedoms, ditch the baby listening monitors at the usual stage and simply trust that their child would pass through all the milestones of childhood and grow safely into adulthood without something bad happening to them.

When You Choose
Not to Have Another Baby

*'We're too scared to try again. Too scared another loss would
break us. It hurts. We'd love another child, not to replace the
ones we've lost but because we feel our home isn't full yet.
We've tried, but the IVF hasn't worked. We're doing our best.
For some of us a rainbow baby isn't coming.'*

Natalie, bereaved mum

Experiencing the death of a baby whom you dearly wanted and
loved does not mean that you will automatically want to try to
have another baby. Equally, you may decide not to have another
baby straight away but to try again later. If you're feeling unsure,
give yourself enough time and space to consider what is best
for you.

Don't be surprised if you feel unsure for a long time before
making this decision and don't allow anyone to pressure you into
trying again when you are not yet ready. There may be both
adults and children around you who will automatically assume
that you want to have another baby, and this could feel very
painful for you. They will all be grieving in their own way and
perhaps feel that another baby would help their own grief. And
while this might be true for them, you are under no obligation
to meet others' expectations, or to help others cope with their
grief. You also do not have to find a reason such as ill health or
infertility to explain why you are not trying to have another baby.

You may want to take the time you need to grieve for the
baby who has died and to explore with those supporting you
how you feel as a parent towards that baby, rather than thinking

about any future parenting. You might also not want to experience any risks and complications that you had with the baby who died, or any health problems that you might have developed as a result of being pregnant. In addition to these concerns, you might not want to risk future loss. The thought of future loss can feel very frightening.

If you don't want another baby but your partner does, try to resolve this as you would any other issue in your relationship. The death of a baby has a huge impact on both of you and so you might find it helpful to arrange couples' therapy to help you talk through some of your feelings and to explore the impact of the loss on your relationship and the ways you can navigate through that impact together.

For the partner who does want another baby, having this denied can feel like a further loss. For them, it can be important to find a way to say goodbye to the baby who has died but also to those babies they imagined they might have. If you have had IVF, there might be embryos remaining. Deciding not to have another baby can feel especially difficult and cause conflict as these embryos could be implanted. It might be possible to donate the embryos for use by other people or for research if you wish, however, this may still create feelings of loss that will need to be processed. Your IVF clinicians will be able to discuss options with you.

Part of #BabyLossAwareness is about trying to help people understand that for a bereaved parent baby loss is something they will carry with them forever.

It will change how they look at things. It will temper the joy they feel with an undercurrent of sadness as they see the children of those around them (or even their own) reach the milestones their lost babies never will.

It has no time limit, no expiration date. It will change how they look at things.

When You Can't Have Another Baby

Not all bereaved parents will have the option of trying to have another baby. Sometimes there are medical or personal reasons why another pregnancy is not possible, such as the mother's health, age or the couple's relationship. Parents who had IVF, for example, will also need to decide whether they are able to bear the emotional and financial costs of going through this process again.

In these situations, it is best to think about where you can get support. Attending a support group for parents who have experienced the death of a baby might be useful in many ways; however, there might also be parents who announce that they are expecting another baby. This can create feelings of jealousy and anger and may provoke an even deeper sense of loss.

The grief of wanting another baby and knowing that this is not possible can compound the feelings of loss for the baby who has just died and, in these circumstances, working on a one-to-one basis with a counsellor who can support you through this grief can be more helpful than attending a group. Some Sands groups have been set up specifically for those parents who are expecting another baby, thereby allowing other groups to support parents solely through their experience of loss. The important thing is to know that you have options to explore so you can find the one that is right for you. The Sands Bereavement Support Team is hugely experienced in supporting parents in all the different situations that can follow the death of a baby including the challenge of trying – or not trying – again. And the online community provides an opportunity to share experiences and ideas with other parents in similar situations and in a non-judgemental way.

CHAPTER 13

The Future

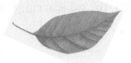

'For an otherwise healthy baby to die undelivered near term is, with hindsight, an easily avoidable event. Research to make it avoidable in practice is a priority.'

Professor Jim Thornton, Professor of Obstetrics
and Gynaecology, University of Nottingham

The primary reason bereaved parents find their way to Sands is because they want and need emotional support, followed by concerns about getting pregnant again and wanting advice about how to handle the grief of existing children. And while the majority asking for such support contact the charity within the first six months of the bereavement, often within the first month, a not insignificant number of parents turn up five or more years after their baby has died.

According to the charity's 2018/19 Annual Impact Report, Sands supported close to 5000 bereaved parents over that 12-month period with more than 2000 of those joining the Sands online community. The majority of calls to the Sands helpline over this 12-month period of analysis were made by parents within the first two months of their baby dying, but some 8 per cent were made by parents whose baby had died over 20 years ago, which speaks volumes as to the total lack of support available following stillbirth or miscarriage to parents less than a generation ago.

Giving Something Back

Many bereaved parents will channel their grief into helping others and by raising funds for Sands to both finance research and campaign for better maternity services, bereavement support for all parents whose baby dies, and greater awareness of the scale of the problem.

One way bereaved parents volunteer is by becoming a 'befriender'. Jen Coates, Director of Bereavement Support and Volunteering at the charity, says, 'Wanting to give back is a beautiful way to create a legacy for a baby who has died, but we have to be sure someone is ready for their sake, as well as for those they may be supporting. We hold fast to our selection criteria and the key skillset we know Befrienders need to be able to offer. So both the interview process and the Befriender training are about self-awareness, and developing those skills of active listening and being able to hold the space for other bereaved parents.'

Sands is also taking steps now to broaden the volunteer opportunities so that as well as training Befrienders who want to support within a support group, they are training others who want to support through, for example, the Sands United initiative (see page 109).

Italian-born Gigliola Hartley, who shares her story below, says her volunteer work as a Sands Befriender – helping other bereaved parents and educating healthcare professionals – gives the death of her baby daughter, Livia, meaning.

LIVIA: BORN 12 AUGUST 2010

My name is Gigliola and my husband is Matt (I think only his mum calls him Matthew!). We got married thirteen years ago after three years of a long-distance relationship while I was in Italy, where I'm from, and Matt was living in London. After the first year of marriage, we decided to start trying for a baby. At the time we lived in Loughton, Essex, and I worked as a primary school teacher in Epping.

For more than a year I couldn't get pregnant, so the GP referred us to have some tests. At my scan, it was discovered that I have a uterus didelphys (better known as a double uterus), which means that the chances of getting pregnant naturally were 50/50. After another year of trying to have a baby and sorting out an infection caused by an operation aimed to improve the functionality of my uterus, we were finally referred to have IVF treatment. At the time we moved to Hertford, in Hertfordshire, and I was still commuting to Epping to teach.

In January 2010 we had our first treatment. We knew our chances of getting pregnant at the first attempt were slim, so we were not very hopeful. We had ICSI (which is slightly different from IVF because the sperm is injected directly into the nucleus of the egg). As a result of the ICSI, ten embryos were produced of which only one carried on growing. This was the embryo that was transferred to my womb. We had no real hopes it would work, but we were still hoping that this embryo would be strong enough to become our baby. To our surprise, I found out I was pregnant with that embryo which we straight away started to call 'Bean'.

Because of my uterus, the chances of growth restriction and risk of stillbirth were high, so I was classified as a high-risk pregnancy and, after 20 weeks, started having scans every 2 weeks. All was proceeding well (I only had a bleed at 21/22 weeks but that didn't seem to have any explanation) and at the 20-week scan we found out we were going to have a girl who we decided to call Livia.

I was keeping a diary about the pregnancy and at about 28 weeks I wrote that the sonographer told me that Livia was not growing a lot but, although in the lowest percentile, there was no concern, so I was just left to hope she would have picked up a bit more weight by the time I had the next scan. At the 30-week scan, this time the sonographer (a different one every time) told me that not only had Livia not gained a lot more weight but she asked me if I had a family history of small heads, as Livia's head was a bit on the small side.

A different registrar consultant (again every time a different consultant, who likely didn't read any of my notes as I constantly had to remind them of my double uterus, the majority of whom didn't even know what it meant) told me that they were slightly concerned about Livia's growth but as she was still on the borderline of the lower percentile, they didn't think they needed to take any action . . . that day they sent me home just asking me to count the movements . . . the consultant told me that there were meant to be at least 10 a day.

Livia had a little pattern. She was fully awake during the day and she slept through the night waking up at about 6am, so she was my natural alarm clock. She did her first 10 movements within the first hour of being awake in the morning, so as far as I was concerned, she was OK, therefore I didn't pay much attention to her movements during the rest of the day.

On the Sunday morning of 8 August 2010 Livia didn't wake up as usual. I prodded her to wake her up, but nothing. Only a few hours later, when I still couldn't feel her and thought it wasn't normal, I called the hospital. They asked me to go in to be checked. On the way there my husband and I didn't speak as if, deep down, we knew, but were of course still hopeful.

The midwife couldn't find the heartbeat but didn't say anything. She went to call one of the consultants available who brought in a portable scan and after a few minutes very bluntly said: 'I'm sorry, your baby is dead.'

I'll never forget those moments and those words. They were like many swords going in my heart all of a sudden.

After the initial cry with my husband, my first reaction was to have her out, but the doctor persuaded me that the best thing to do was to deliver her naturally. Despite hating him for breaking the news, I need to thank him because he avoided me having to have a major operation involving more physical pain, but mainly this allowed me to say goodbye to my baby girl. I was sent home and the next day the process of induction started and after four days, on Thursday the 12th at 1pm, Livia was born with just two pushes but a lot of gas and air and morphine.

Because of the morphine I was asleep for many hours. My husband, who helped the midwife to clean and dress Livia, tried to wake me up a few times to give me the chance to see and to hold her. Sadly, I was totally knocked out so couldn't remember much of her while I was awake. When I actually started to be awake, at about 11pm, Livia had already started to deteriorate and wasn't looking as beautifully sleeping anymore, so we had to say goodbye. I so much regret taking so much morphine, but no one told me what it would have meant and sadly we couldn't rely on cuddle cold cots which didn't exist yet.

My parents had flown over from Italy the day after we told them Livia had died (they wanted, of course, to support us). My mum stayed with us during the delivery, struggling with the different methods used in the UK. While my dad stayed at home, watching over us from the distance. I was cross with him as he refused to see Livia. He admitted that in his mind he thought he would have seen a little monster. Only when I was back home, after Livia had gone, I showed her pictures to my dad. She looked as a beautiful girl sleeping. He then realised what he had missed.

I didn't seek help straight away. I thought it was my grief

to deal with and I needed to be strong, but I couldn't. My husband wasn't crying with me every day, then he went back to work after a few weeks and to me he looked like he had 'moved on' but I didn't want to, and I wondered why he behaved as if nothing had happened. I then learned to understand he grieves in a different way.

I was a primary school teacher and I had left my school at the end of the school year heavily pregnant thinking that not only would I have taken a year's maternity leave, but that I'd have actually left my job and become a full-time mum teaching my own child. After losing Livia, it destroyed me; the thought of having to come back to work teaching other children, in an environment I didn't particularly like and with two of my colleagues who had given birth in August to healthy babies. I decided to leave my job and change my career.

In the meantime, as I couldn't find any comfort and was alone (we had just moved to Hertford, so I didn't know anyone), I decided to seek help from Sands. That was my saviour. I found that I wasn't going mad and I wasn't the only one feeling in a certain way.

I then spoke to the vicar of the church that my husband rigorously attended every Sunday (his way to find comfort) to ask if I could volunteer doing whatever to keep myself occupied. He told me about a Nigerian lady who started a business of cake-making and told me that she had lost her first child having to terminate the pregnancy at 16 weeks (who therefore could understand my pain) and that she needed help with her business. I started to go to her house every day, spending most of the day there and really enjoyed helping her and her company. I guess she helped me to relax a little and I'm convinced that helped me to become pregnant naturally with my rainbow baby, Alex.

Times got better but there was a lot of anxiety and comparisons with Livia. I didn't want another child to replace Livia. I always wanted and still wish Livia could be here.

Alex was born, with lots of blues and an incredible sense of protection. Despite the fears of losing another baby, we wanted to give Alex another brother or sister so, again naturally, after three years I got pregnant with another baby, another boy, Marcus.

Sands has helped me enormously and I felt that I needed to do something to make the death of Livia somehow meaningful. I therefore decided to become a Befriender and, for three years now, I've been running the East Herts Sands group, which gives me at the same time sadness knowing that still so many babies die and therefore many families are affected by this horrible pain, but also hope to help grieving parents get those tools . . . opening up, talking about their baby, making memories, dealing with others who don't understand how to deal with grief. I also work with the hospitals to make sure that all the parents going through the same get the best care in and outside the hospital.'

THE IMPORTANCE OF SELF-CARE

It feels good to be needed and to help others in their time of need, but there's a delicate balance between being the one everyone can count on to park their own feelings and 'be there' in that difficult empathic space and taking care of your own feelings through the process.

There are those who take the view a wound can't heal if you keep picking at the scab, but the wounds left when a baby dies – and the ongoing injuries caused when you try to pick up those shattered shards of mirror to put together a new version of yourself – are going to leave scars, whether you pick the scab or not.

Lots of the bereaved parents who have contributed to this book are heavily involved with Sands, taking on both supportive and campaigning roles to raise awareness of the charity's work and the challenges facing any family whose baby dies, but who looks after the Befrienders? And how can they be sure taking such an active role is not a subconscious way of trying to side-step the terrific and ongoing onslaught of grief that won't go away by looking the other way?

Befriender Pete Byrom, who won a Sands Volunteer of the Year award in 2019, admitted in a blog he wrote at the end of what had been a very difficult year for him that his work for and with Sands had been a welcome and actively-sought distraction from the death of his father that year, and that it was only when his doctor signed him off work with a diagnosis of stress and anxiety that he was able to admit he wasn't coping and was being (his words) 'a dumbass' in not following his own advice to other bereaved families.

One of the triggers for finding himself struggling to be 'Pete from Sands' and the one everyone turned to for help was that he and his wife, Denise, were making regular trips to a hospital for her to have dialysis treatment (their home machine had broken down) which was right opposite the maternity unit where their first son, Thomas, had been stillborn 14 years earlier (see page 182 for Pete's story).

'It was probably the closest we'd been to returning to "the scene of the crime",' Pete writes in his blog. 'I realised it had subconsciously been piling on top of everything else and once I realised that was what had been getting to me, I thought that was it. Just by recognising it I'd dealt with it. Like I said, I was a dumbass.'

Any additional bereavement is going to plunge someone back into the place where they are still grieving the death of their baby, no matter how much time has passed. But it wasn't until his worried wife, Denise, posted this on Facebook that Pete let go of the floodgates, started the grieving process for his father, found a place for it alongside his grief over the death of Thomas, and took himself off to the doctor to get the help he needed.

Denise had written: 'So proud of my husband whose commitment to Sands is constant and who always carries on trying to help others – regardless of the grief he feels – especially following the loss of his father this year and the loss of our son which is always in his mind and heart. Peter – I know while you seem externally to be fine you need to be kind to yourself and ask for support and understanding when you need it and share your feelings – others assume you are there for them but do not think of you as they are thinking only of themselves – grief is a selfish mistress.'

'Ten minutes later, when I finished crying, I realised I needed to do something,' recalls Pete. 'I thought I was clever enough to either deal with all the emotions of the last few months when I was ready or that I could get past them altogether. I'd read what the symptoms of anxiety and depression are. I'd recognised them in myself. I just thought I could live with them, but I was wrong.'

Lifting the Carpet

Sadly, the death of a baby, as we have seen throughout this book, is not a rare event: currently around 14 babies die before, during or soon after birth every day in the UK. In 2018, 1 in every 250 births was a stillbirth; 1 in every 360 babies died within the first 4 weeks of life.

Loving You From Here is published to coincide with the fifth annual Baby Loss Awareness Week, which is a collaborative campaign between some 60-plus baby loss charities around the UK that form the Baby Loss Awareness Alliance Group (www.babylossawareness.org). The campaign, led by Sands, gives parents, their families and their friends an opportunity to acknowledge and remember their babies who have died, and is also designed to raise awareness about the issues surrounding pregnancy and baby loss in the UK and push for tangible improvements in bereavement care and support. The initiative has also been instrumental in the UK government now acknowledging one of society's last great taboos – talking about the death of a baby – by holding its own annual debate on the subject to mark the start of Baby Loss Awareness Week each year.

In 2018, the then Minister for Care, Caroline Dinenage, welcomed what was the fourth Baby Loss Awareness Week debate with the following words: 'This debate helps to send a clear signal outside this place about the importance of this subject in the Chamber, in the Department of Health and Social Care and in the National Health Service.

'Over the years, many Members of Parliament have been brave enough to share their own personal and painful accounts of baby loss which, while heartbreaking to hear, have done so much to raise the profile of this important issue and to start vital conversations about it. It is absolutely right and fundamentally important that we continue to raise awareness of both the devastating impact of baby loss and the support that bereaved parents need through the grieving process to help them adjust to their loss.

'I do not think people ever fully heal or get over the loss of a much-loved and much-wanted child, but with the right care and support they might be able slowly to move forward with their lives.'

Pulling no punches, Mr Jim Cunningham, the now retired but then Labour MP for Coventry South, supported the Minister's opening remarks adding: 'It has been very good to have these debates because they educate the public about an issue that has too often been "shoved under the carpet", for want of a better term.'

Our vision is for a world where fewer babies die and when a baby does die, anyone affected receives the best possible care and support for as long as it is needed.

Sands UK Mission Statement

SUPPORTING RESEARCH

Since 2010, the Sands research fund has invested close to £1 million, supporting some 20 different projects, many of which focus, in some way, on finding answers to the question 'Why are our babies still dying?' and, as a result, helping reduce the numbers of babies dying in the UK; with others exploring what can make a positive difference to the experience of parents when the worst happens and their baby dies.

Past studies have looked at how to use scans to predict the risk of a baby's death towards the end of pregnancy, how foetal monitoring of baby's movements might reduce the risk of stillbirth, post-mortem practices in order to challenge current thinking about what investigations give the best information, and to hear from bereaved parents about their experiences of consenting to autopsy and how culture and religion play a part in that decision. Another study explored the economic cost of stillbirth.

Ongoing live projects include looking at outcomes when resuscitation efforts extend beyond the normal 10 minutes (after which they are traditionally stopped), how pregnant women use digital platforms to identify 'red flags' during pregnancy, and how doctors working on the neonatal intensive care unit (NICU) can benefit from specialised training around end-of-life and the palliative care of babies who will die.

The Midlands and North of England Stillbirth Study, co-funded by Sands, found that pregnant women who sleep on their side in the last trimester of pregnancy are less likely to have a stillborn baby. This advice is now shared on the saferpregnancy.org.uk website.

Over the last five years, the charity has also been involved in numerous NHS initiatives, including the NHS England Saving Babies' Lives care bundle which specifies four interventions aimed at helping healthcare professionals improve care in pregnancy and labour to prevent stillbirths. In 2019 a second version of the Care Bundle was launched, which included an additional element to reduce preterm birth. In an evaluation of 19 participating units, researchers found a 20 per cent reduction in the number of stillbirths between 2013 and 2017.

These interventions include giving advice about quitting smoking during pregnancy; monitoring foetal growth and movement; monitoring the baby during labour; and listening carefully when mothers report concerns about their baby's reduced movements in the womb.

'With stillbirth research in its early days, it's vital to build up a strong body of evidence. Roughly 3,000 papers have currently been published on the subject and no comprehensive review of active research studies has yet been undertaken. Small pockets of research have been taking place which can't be translated on a national scale. For example, no standard guidance on what clinicians should do when women report *reduced foetal movements exists yet because there's a lack of evidence on what works best.'*

From 'The Stillbirth Priority Setting Partnership'
report

Change is Happening . . .

'For many years cancer was talked about in hushed tones and was stigmatised. This is no longer the case. If we can raise awareness of stillbirth and neonatal death, we reduce isolation and go some way to acknowledging families' grief, creating a positive legacy for all the babies who have sadly died.'

Jen Coates, Director of Bereavement Support
and Volunteering, Sands

By sharing their stories of grief, growth and hope throughout this book, bereaved parents – especially those, like David and Julia Haig (see page 205), whose baby died less recently – know that change is slow, but it is happening, and Dr Clea Harmer, CEO of Sands, echoes those hopeful sentiments:

'In every single one of the three areas we work in – research and prevention, improving bereavement care, and bereavement support – there are opportunities and change is happening. There is a very real hope we can make some of the changes that need to be made. We can never take the pain away when a baby dies, and we can never stop every baby dying, but we can make it so much better for every parent and, as a charity, we can do so much more.

I feel I am so lucky to have this opportunity to get out there and make a difference. It is a real privilege to have this role, which is one of service to enable everyone else to do the brilliant job they do in Sands.'

CHAPTER 14

Loving You
From Here

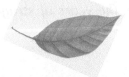

'Out of suffering have emerged the strongest souls;
the most massive characters are seared with scars.'

From *The Broken Wings* by Kahlil Gibran

The love, which will have started as soon as you made space in
your mind and in your life for a baby, a new person to love,
does not die. But where is 'Here'? It's an ethereal concept and
place – often mercurial too – that will mean different things to
different parents, depending on which stage of the challenge of
growing around grief and forming an enduring bond with their
baby they find themselves.

At the start of that challenge, the shock, grief and disbelief
will likely overwhelm any sense of place other than the hinter-

land (the place of immense shock and grief described in Chapter 1) those bereaved by the death of a baby, an infant, a miscarriage or an ectopic pregnancy find themselves banished to. But 'Here' is a destination all bereaved parents can and must reach.

Ethereal, yes, and as such, beautiful too. Like the ethereal senescence of a quiet winter garden. You have had or may still have a mountain to climb to get 'Here' but just look at the view when you do, both inwardly (who you have become) and outwardly (how you have become).

'One day, in retrospect, the years of struggle will strike you as the most beautiful.'

Sigmund Freud

Fiona Gilmour is a London-based, Australian-born art psychotherapist whose baby daughter, Aphra Milli McMahon, died on 15 June 1993. Six months later, Fiona was pregnant with her son, Finn, who is now in his mid-twenties. When I met Fiona, who specialises in bereavement and grief, and invited her to contribute to this book, she sent me some writing so powerful I knew I wanted to share it, unadulterated by me and in its entirety. For those of us now decades on from the death of our babies, we share her understanding of the 'Here' place and of actively loving the babies we did not get to bring home with us.

For those still growing around their grief, she captures the essence of this ethereal but inspirational place when she describes how she has worked hard to transform a 'spiral of grief' so wretched it was the darkest place she had ever been into gifts that have since nourished her own life and the lives of others; thanks, she says, entirely to her ongoing love for Aphra.

APHRA MILLI MCMAHON: BORN 15 JUNE 1993

Aphra was my first baby with my then-partner Alan McMahon. I was 33 years old and he was 46 and at that time we were living in Kentish Town in North London. When I discovered I was pregnant, I was both surprised and completely over the moon – she wasn't planned and yet she wasn't not planned. I was at a huge crossroad in my life – searching for both meaning and direction – so it made perfect sense to be pregnant and embrace Motherhood as a complete embodied soul journey, sensing that she had found her way to me as much as I to her.

Throughout the pregnancy all went well. I was healthy and happy and excited to learn and embrace all the knowledge available to me. I read books, went swimming and talked a lot to other women. I joined a prenatal yoga group which became like my surrogate family.

The prenatal yoga group was run by a wonderful teacher and was attended by an amazing circle of women in all stages of pregnancy. We not only did yoga together, but we shared stories of our week; progress of our baby's health and growth, as well as our hopes and fears. We knew when each one of us went into labour – coming back to the group with her baby, to share all the minutiae of their birth story. It was here I learned that birth has its own timeframe and its journey from start to finish can meander way off the planned and hoped-for course.

But, so far, in this small tribe of North London women, there was always a baby to see and hold at the end . . .

For all my research, I strangely never gave one moment's thought that my baby or any baby might die.

As a result of going to the yoga group, Alan and I decided we wanted to have a home birth within the NHS. Throughout the pregnancy Aphra was in a breech position and by 34 weeks she still hadn't turned into the preferred cephalic position for a natural birth. The NHS obstetrician told me that if at 36 weeks she was still breech they would perform an external cephalic version (ECV). The same doctor also said that if, when doing the procedure, Aphra started to show any signs of distress they would do an emergency caesarean.

At the end of that meeting I suddenly felt as if I'd been thrown into a cold, clinical, matter-of-fact, male world of obstetrics and procedures. I felt very anxious and confused.

I then spoke with my yoga teacher and we discussed other ways to try to get Aphra to turn from being breech. This included acupuncture as well as lying upside down on an ironing board trying to encourage her to do this watery somersault naturally.

At the same time, I decided to transfer my care to a group of independent midwives, primarily because the NHS home birth team consisted of a team of five or more midwives, most of whom I hadn't met, plus I had no guarantee of knowing who would come on the day. I felt it was important to have some consistency of care from one or two midwives whom I'd met.

The plan of care we agreed to was part-private, part-NHS, meaning that if I needed to be transferred to hospital, I would go to my local NHS hospital, but all other care, such as monitoring in pregnancy, would happen in the private hospital where the independent midwives worked.

At 36 weeks, Aphra still hadn't turned and it was arranged for me to meet with a private obstetrician and have her turned by a private sonographer. This was done and all seemed well with Aphra remaining head down.

The weeks went by, I passed 40 weeks but still no sign of labour starting. I was told this was quite normal for a woman having her first baby and we would wait and see a little longer. At 42 weeks, Alan and I went to the private hospital to have Aphra monitored and were pleased that the labour had started naturally.

I was attached to the monitor, which was showing signs of deceleration in Aphra's heart rate and the midwife suggested that I spend some time in the Jacuzzi to relax before being put back on the monitor. She concluded that everything was fine and told us to go home.

As Alan and I were leaving the hospital my waters broke and I saw that there was a pea soup discharge – meconium. I was anxious and went back to see the midwife. She looked at the meconium, explaining that there were different 'grades' indicated by the meconium's texture, colour and the stage of labour, saying it wasn't unusual, there was nothing to worry about and that the NHS would overreact. She suggested we go home, saying she'd be with me in a couple of hours.

When the midwife arrived, my contractions were very strong, and I thought all was going well but after several attempts in between strong contractions she couldn't find Aphra's heartbeat. She immediately called an ambulance to transfer me to my NHS hospital where it was confirmed that my darling daughter had died.

I then spent several days in hospital and finally gave birth to Aphra via caesarean section. In the days that followed I held her and took photographs of the three of us together. My state of mind was total bewilderment. I remember looking at her, thinking she just seems to be asleep and that she would wake up any minute.

There is so much more to say here about the early months and first year following Aphra's death. My grief was the most wretched spiral into the deepest darkness I'd ever imagined.

The NHS needed to know why Aphra died, which resulted in an enquiry and a legal case taken out against the midwife, since such a catalogue of misjudgements and errors had been made. The investigation resulted in the first midwife being suspended and her partner decided to stop practicing.

At the same time this grief-stricken battle of accountability was going on, I got pregnant with my adorable son, Finn, who is always my life's blessing alongside his big sister. This is a card written by me to Alan from Aphra on her first anniversary, a month before Finn was born:

To My Dear Dad,

Today is my first-year anniversary and I wanted to tell you how much I love you and to tell you that I am always with you . . . sometimes I hide in your pocket, and sometimes I walk along with you, holding your hand, and sometimes I give you little kisses on your cheek . . . I'm always there and always here . . . wherever you go . . .

And, I love it best of all when you talk to me about how you feel and what you're thinking about . . .

I just love you very much ~ because I am your bright purple star . . .

Aphra Milli McMahon xxx

Fiona told me that when she wrote her story for this book, it felt as if it had all happened yesterday. She was right back in the pain of that experience; not as raw, but painful, nonetheless. Here then, again in her own words, are her final thoughts about the place – 'Here' – from where she is still so actively loving her baby daughter and encouraging the rest of us to do the same.

It is now 26 years since Aphra died and I feel her story is important to tell because of the enormous unwavering love that I have for her and that, through this love, I have been able to transform my unbearable grief into gifts that hopefully continue to nourish myself and others.

My heart broke open to reveal more than I could have imagined – namely a voice and desire to break the silence surrounding a mother's grief.

Going home with empty arms was the worst imaginable feeling – I couldn't leave my flat for weeks – facing neighbours and people in the local community who had watched my belly growing; wishing me well and saying 'not long now . . .'

My partner, Alan, had to take over with all the practicalities of life. That was tough.

I want my story to honour him and all the other fathers whose voices and experiences often get lost. They carry the burden of facing the outside world on behalf of the mother – this is their great strength.

All my immediate family live in Australia, so I felt very alone, relying on good friends to listen and hold my pain. I learned too how hard it is for a lot of people to know what to say to a grieving mother for fear of upsetting her.

Unfortunately, this is the worst misunderstanding ever as you're left to manage the awkwardness of others' feelings as well as your own pain.

I hope the writing of this book can really challenge and change this misunderstanding – any words of condolence, no matter how uncomfortable, are always better than none.

Six months after Aphra died I became pregnant with my son Finn. For me, I could see no other path ahead than to be a mother. I would love Aphra's story to honour and validate Finn's loss too, and all the children who have lost a sibling, for even though he never met her, she is his sister and she has shaped so much of the family lens that we see life through.

At this time, I also started my own journey of personal therapy and, when Finn was three, I joined a ceramics class for one day a week and found that, completely unexpectedly, the clay allowed me to mould my grief into forms that held meaning and beauty. This led me on to studying Art Psychotherapy and I have been practicing ever since.

Aphra's life brought me the gift of using the creative process in all its forms to transform and find meaning in the unbearable. *Bearing the Unbearable* is the name of a beautiful book by Joanne Cacciatore, which explores 'love, loss and the heartbreaking path of grief'. This has become a phrase I often use with clients in my psychotherapy practice, for that's what losing Aphra has come to be: a journey of bearing a pain so deeply incomprehensible and transforming it into a palpable, alive form that has words, substance and hope.

In the bewilderment of my grief I saw an almost imperceptible thread where the anticipation of life meets the ground of death almost in the same moment – the two sides are just a tiny hair's breadth apart. Paradoxically, I feel that every woman who loses a baby is a testimony to honouring life.

For those in any doubt about the impact our dead children have, however many years since they died, Fiona sums it up beautifully when she says: 'These babies, they find us too and keep coming and tapping on our shoulders saying I have something for you to do. So, for me, the phrase "loving you from here" says it all.

'I am loving Aphra from another dimension and that "here" place is my heart, and my work, and my emotions and everything I think, say and do. Until Aphra died, and Finn was born, I didn't realise how precious life was. So, I guess the place from where we are loving these babies is this ongoing life place.'

This makes perfect sense to those of us who have had that gift of time that bereaved dad, David Haig, describes on page 205 to help us grow around the grief and sorrow of our baby dying, but when that first happens, and even a year or two after, the feelings can be so raw still that it may feel we will never be able to make this kind of peace with our loss.

This is when, more than at any other time, we need to trust the words and wisdom of those who have walked this way before us when they tell us if they did it – found the place from where we can still love and cherish our baby who died, but also grow around our grief and find a new normal – then please trust that you will too.

'So, either I've been dreaming about Sylvie,' I said to myself, 'or this is the reality. Or else I've really been with Sylvie, and this is a dream! Is life itself a dream, I wonder?'

From *Sylvie and Bruno*, Lewis Carroll, 1889

Over lunch, at the 2019 Sands conference which was held in London, I sat on a small wooden bench placed alongside the wall and noticed that the woman at the other end of the bench was upset and sitting alone. We began to speak and, as she explained she had travelled down from Scotland to attend the conference, I noticed too that she had a small tattoo with the name 'Sylvie-Rose' on the inside of her left wrist. I remember thinking what a pretty name she had chosen for the daughter who, she began to tell me, had died in utero and it struck me just how palpable her love for that child was because, simply by chatting with her, I could feel the strength and depth of it.

Janine explained she was alone because her husband had taken their children (born subsequently) Rory, now six, and Adara, now four, to the Natural History Museum for the day. My heart just went out to Janine. She was so dignified in her sorrow for her little girl and I understood something important about the idea of 'loving you from here', namely it is a commitment you make to your baby who died. It is a choice; a loving, a humbling and a courageous one.

Janine asked me the name of my baby/babies and I squirmed, because, until this point, I had not given myself – or, looking back – anyone else permission to love my children from anywhere. It was a topic my therapist had raised with me over and over once I had started talking about the babies; my guilt over what he called their 'two deaths' – their physical death at birth and then a second death in the way I had refused to allow them to matter and to be acknowledged. And, although I had agreed to write this book almost 12 months before meeting Janine, it was her conversation with me over that lunch break that finally connected me to what 'loving you from here' meant for bereaved parents setting out from the hinterland, along with grief and then hoping to find a new place from which to do just that.

SYLVIE-ROSE: BORN 1 FEBRUARY 2013

We found out we were expecting on 3 August 2012, the day before my thirty-first birthday. To say we were delighted is an understatement. The pregnancy progressed well; she was wriggly and had a strong heartbeat. On 31 January 2013, I went in for my 28-week check-up.

There was no heartbeat.

Our little girl had died in utero.

Our world fell apart.

The next day we went into the hospital so I could be induced. She came into this world, silently, at 2:45pm weighing 1lb 11.5 and measuring 32cm. She was beautiful and perfect, and we exclaimed over her as any new parents would.

So much has been taken from us; our dreams and hopes for Sylvie-Rose. We'll never know if she was fiery with my sense of adventure or calm, quiet, patient and gentle like her daddy.

We can only try to focus on the joy and love she brought to our life. From the moment we found out we were expecting, we were ecstatic, and each milestone brought new happiness, wonder and contentment. Telling our families and friends, the first scan, the first movement.

The first time Callum felt Sylvie-Rose kick was the most

joyous moment of our lives. We wish we could have kept her, but we know she's waiting for us, beyond the stars. We're trying to make her legacy one of joy and transformation.

Sylvie and Bruno is a book by Lewis Carroll I read several years ago and I loved the name Sylvie from that moment on. Sylvie means 'of the forest' and is ethereal and delicate as was our Sylvie girl when she was born. Roses are my favourite flower and remind me of my wedding dress and my gran's garden. When we saw her, we knew her name had to be Sylvie-Rose.

With her beautiful rosebud pout, she was the bonniest lass we have ever seen.

It is love that will keep us going through the dark days. Our love for each other, our love from our families and the love from our friends.

'Loving you from here' is a commitment bereaved parents make to their baby who died. Some parents run marathons and climb mountains to make sure the memory of their baby stays alive, while others adopt private rituals that maintain the love and their link with their dead child.

Janine, who is currently the chair of the Fife Sands support group, has a tattoo of her daughter's name on her left wrist because, she explains, that's closer to the heart than the right wrist, and it is also done in purple ink which fades, to represent the fading of the pain.

Making that commitment to loving your dead baby from here – and nurturing your enduring bond with them as a result – is, Janine says, the single biggest thing you can do to find your way back to joy and happiness, without forgetting the baby who died.

It also, she admits in her continuing story below, might just sneak up on you because you are making that supreme effort.

If you had told me at the time Sylvie-Rose died that I would ever laugh again, or love again, or feel confident again, I would never have believed you. The joy goes out of life and you feel like you'll never be able to do the things again that you took for granted before. I felt that way for a really, really long time.

I started to feel better once my wee boy, Rory, who's now six, was out of the woods after his illness. When he was born, he was in intensive care for the first four weeks of his life. He had two operations, was very poorly, and the doctors kept telling us he might not make it. I was planning his funeral as well; I thought well that's what happens to me, my babies die. But he defied all expectations and now you would never know.

The day after we got him home, some close friends were getting married and so we decided to surprise them and go. It was a fantastic day – the bride didn't see us until she was walking down the aisle, at which point, she promptly burst into tears.

It was wonderful showing off my new baby, but it was bittersweet too because I was getting to show my boy off and saying look at this beautiful baby but, at the same time, I was thinking I should have my girl here to show her off as well.

We'd gone along to a Sands support group about five months after Sylvie-Rose died and so, by the time I was pregnant with Rory, we were going to the Trying Again group and I managed to get some counselling through my GP as well while I was pregnant.

But it was a really, really hard time. In the latter half of the pregnancy, I barely left the house. I was really just in a dark place. I didn't like to go out without Callum and if we did go out, I didn't want to see anyone I knew. We ended up visiting a lot of remote castles because I just didn't want to deal with other people at all.

I didn't go out during the week, except to go and sit on Sylvie-Rose's bench; I'd go and sit there by myself with a book and a cup of tea. I needed a lot of time on my own. I watched a lot of box sets and read a lot of books which was pure escapism and trying to live other people's lives, so I didn't have to think about my own.

It literally was just one day at a time; one hospital meeting at a time.

There's no question that Rory, one thousand per cent, brought the light back to our lives. He brought the joy back. Life does carry on and, if it doesn't, you're not honouring your little one that died. This is how I do it. I live the biggest and best life that I can because Sylvie-Rose didn't get to do that; so, I need to live it for her and do whatever I can to make the world maybe a little bit easier and happier for other people.

I remember going along to the Sands group where other parents had gone on to deliver babies and were going on nights out and dancing again and I was thinking how can they do that? And now I'm the one doing that.

It's as if the joy snuck back up on me because of Rory –

just the absolute wonder and awe of a new baby; there are no words that can describe it, and seeing the world through his eyes and him laughing at things which would make me laugh, but it was also a decision on my part to be happy again.

I was watching him one day and just burst into tears because I was thinking about Sylvie-Rose and then I thought I've got to make sure he has a happy life and make sure that everything I had planned for her happens for him. I realised it's not fair for him to have his life overcast by the shadow of a dead sister.

For example, I had always loved Christmas and gone all out, but the first Christmas after Sylvie-Rose died, I couldn't face it and the following one, which was Rory's first Christmas, having just come out of hospital I couldn't face it again. But the next year I thought no, we're doing this and we're doing it properly. Same for his first birthday – we went all out and had a party and took him on a little day trip.

We always celebrate Sylvie-Rose's birthday too; we make a cake and take flowers to her bench in the park. And this year, which would have been her seventh birthday, Rory said he wanted balloons for her too. His little sister, Adara, who's now four, also talks about Sylvie-Rose. They both know who she is.

It's difficult to see any hope at the start when your baby dies, but it does come. Being involved with Sands really helped restore my confidence and doing all that charity work helped me get back in the job market. I think we hide that loss of confidence that follows the death of your baby, we put the face on, and people think you're fine, but it took me a long time to lift my head again.

It's been stepping-stones and lots of little steps to build my life back up again.

All the bereaved parents who, like Janine, have shared their stories for this book have found a way to love their baby from Here and you will too. It will take time, it may feel as if you will never get Here, but you will, if you want to. As Janine says, little steps . . . and lots of them.

Many bereaved parents, like Erica who shared her story in Chapter 5, write loving letters as part of their commitment to loving their child from here, even when decades have gone by. This is the letter Erica found herself writing to Baby Shane while sitting on a train on the day before the thirty-fifth anniversary of his death:

Dear Baby Shane,
Tomorrow, 29 May 2018, it will have been 35 years since you died. Last week there was an advert on TV advertising a new hamburger, limited edition, until the 29 May they said.

The weather person said it's going to be 29 degrees.

At this time of year, the number 29 seems magnified.

I won't go into work tomorrow in honour of you. I will buy your flowers, freesias, they look so pretty and have the most beautiful scent.

Does the pain lessen? No!

My grief has just found a place to settle inside me, but it will never go completely. Like a wound it can be disturbed, knocked like a scab and bleed again.

There are some things that I wish I had done 35 years ago. I wish I could have held you in my arms when you took your last breath. I wish I had bathed you and dressed you in a special outfit.

Things were so different back then and I didn't have any control over what was happening. Leaving hospital without you was one of the hardest, heartbreaking things I have ever had to do in my life. I am so glad that we came back to collect you and take you home.

At home I held you a lot and changed your nappy. I took you downstairs into the street and showed you the night stars. I read you a story while you were in your rocking cradle, one of the Mr Men books – Mr Funny. I remember thinking, if anyone could see me, they would think I was crazy, but now I realise that doing all these things was my way of nurturing you, my way of being your mummy.

Your sisters came upstairs to see their baby brother. They had visited you in hospital on the neonatal unit many times over the eight weeks but were only able to touch your little hands through the many tubes connected to you.

The day of your funeral arrived, and I knew I had to let you go. Your dad and I put you in your coffin and your dad screwed the lid down. I often wonder how we did that. You looked so still, so peaceful, I was no longer scared of death or dying after that. It hurt so much, but at the same time it was an honour and privilege. I remember thinking that there is such a thin line between life and death.

Your dad and I planned and led your funeral by ourselves. I asked everyone to wear white. I felt that this reflected your pureness.

It was hard after your funeral because I couldn't nurture you or do anything for you anymore. Everyone else just carried on with their lives and why shouldn't they, but my world had stopped, and I found it hard to carry on as 'normal', hard to do the simplest everyday tasks. People couldn't see my pain, my grief. I wanted to tell people about you, that my baby had died. Surely the world would stop for a moment, but it just carried on. That felt like torture! But I had to get on with life; caring for your sisters kept me going, and in many ways kept me sane.

I had a strong urge to have another baby, not to replace you, but to fill my empty arms. It didn't happen immediately, so I kind of stopped thinking about it.

Three years later I discovered I was pregnant again, and I was terrified that this baby was going to have the same heart problem and die. I felt totally anxious for the whole nine months, insisting on extra heart scans and check-ups.

Your brother was born, and the doctor said he was fine. It took me quite a few months to trust that he was going to stay. I remember your dad and I poking him sometimes to make sure he was still breathing. The fear of having another baby die was sometimes overwhelming. As your brother grew up, we told him all about you and showed him your memory box. You will always be included, you are part of our family, and will be for many generations to come. My grandchildren, who are your nieces and nephews, all know about you. And they know that the work I do for Sands is because you existed.

You will always be loved and never ever forgotten.
Love Mummy xxx

Everyone Else . . .

We've seen how the act of 'loving you from here' runs through all the stories of grief, growth and hope in this book and what it means for bereaved parents to have their dead baby acknowledged, loved and remembered. And because it's so important for the parents, that means it's important for those who love and support them to do the same if they can.

Karen is Janine's mother and Sylvie-Rose would also have been her very first grandchild. Karen says that she didn't just lose her granddaughter, she lost her eldest daughter too after Sylvie-Rose died and that it took five long years before she saw Janine, who went on to have two more children, laughing once more.

KAREN'S STORY

My husband, Fred, and I had been living in Canada for three years when it happened – the news was horrendous; the guilt and everything about not being here for her and the time it took to get to her.

She had phoned me just a few days before she had gone to the hospital and said she wasn't feeling any movement, so I had tried to reassure her and said, 'Well, you're almost due; the baby's getting bigger so there's not so much room to move,' and I tried to be positive.

The day she went into hospital for a check, her husband was away working so she went in on her own when she was told that the baby's heart wasn't beating any more. I remember she called her younger sister, Ailsa, to come and be with her.

And then we got the phone call.

Because of the time difference, we were still in bed and I knew something was amiss because it was an early morning call.

I think it was Ailsa that called, and she just said, 'Janine has lost the baby.'

I just broke down in tears. I felt like my heart had been ripped out. It was just awful . . .

I know I didn't lose any babies but as a mother, you can put yourself in their shoes and know how you would feel if it was you.

We had kept in touch via video calls and throughout the pregnancy Janine had never looked so happy and glowing in her life. The Christmas before – Sylvie-Rose was stillborn on 1 February – she looked glowing, and I had said that to her. Everybody was devastated. There were no words. I didn't just feel like I'd lost my granddaughter, I felt like I'd lost my daughter as well.

We came back for the funeral and met Sylvie-Rose – she looked just like a little baby doll – but we got to say hello/ goodbye and that made a huge difference. It wasn't that seeing her made her real to me, she was always going to be real, it was the fact we got the chance to speak to her.

I then came back for the month when she would have been born; I'd already booked that flight to come home. I told Janine I was here for her and she could talk to me anytime but if I tried to talk about how I felt, she shut me down because she said she couldn't deal with my feelings.

I think the hardest thing for her was friends and family who, after six months, thought she should be getting over it. They couldn't understand that things would set her off – understandably so – and sometimes even I forget to include Sylvie-Rose as one of her children; I'll say you have two kids and she'll correct me and say I've got three kids.

I know my daughter very well and I could see how angry she was getting with other people and how they were reacting. Everybody deals with grief a different way but it's always there . . . it never goes away . . . but life grows around it and so you do begin to have normality again.

It's really only in the last couple of years my daughter's come back; Christmas 2018 was the first time I saw her laughing and meaning it and not just putting on a front in social surroundings.

I think what really got her through all this has been her involvement in Sands. She went, at first, as a bereaved parent, then she joined the committee and then became the chair of her local branch. She's heavily involved and I'm so proud of her.

I think the way we, as a family, are able to love Sylvie-Rose from here is by making sure we never forget her. We talk openly about her and celebrate her birthday and think about her at Christmas. We've put a bench in the local park so when we want to sit with her, we can; and we take flowers there for her on her birthday and at Christmas. Her little brother and sister know about her and when they see other people sitting there, they say, 'Oh, they're sitting on my sister's bench.'

I think celebrating Sylvie-Rose and talking about her has

helped us all get through; Janine loves people to say her name. She has her name tattooed on the inside of her wrist and both her dad and I have tattoos in Sylvie-Rose's memory too. Mine is on my foot, and he has the heart that Janine talks about from the book, *Sylvie and Bruno*, which inspired Sylvie-Rose's name, and which says, depending which way you read it, 'All will love Sylvie or Sylvie will love all.'

I had mine done the summer after Sylvie-Rose died and Fred had his done a couple of years after that. I had mine on my foot so I can cover it up if I need to but when people see it they say what a beautiful tattoo and then I get to tell them Sylvie-Rose's story.

She will always be there for us, she will always be part of our family. Janine doesn't believe in heaven or God and tells the children Sylvie-Rose is in the stars, but I am quite spiritual, so I like to think she's up there with my mum and dad looking after her.

Your baby's death has changed you. In so many ways. You're no longer imprisoned in the hinterland without the tools to hack out of the fortress of grief and across the thicket of silence. And, as we've seen from the stories bereaved parents have shared throughout the book, it is grief itself which has forced you to grow and travelled with you, a constant companion, as you find a new 'normal'.

It is grief, not hate, that lies on the other side of love; a deep and lasting grief simply reflects the deep and lasting love you have for the child you did not get to keep.

It has not been easy getting Here – nothing worth having is. There has been no magic bullet cure or quick fix and, while going on to have subsequent children surely has an ameliorating effect on your terrible grief and devastation, it is not a cure or a replacement for what you have lost.

This Enduring Bond

Many bereaved parents grow, albeit painfully, into enviable qualities including compassion and empathy; many freely give endless hours to help support other bereaved parents and, just as importantly, raise funds so that things – medical research, government policy – will change, all in the hope that fewer parents will follow behind with the same devastating experience; and, above all this, they are brave. They don't feel brave, they don't know they are brave, but they are. And it is this courage which is inspiring and the quality that means all bereaved parents should be admired, not ignored, shunned or belittled.

They have so much to give.

And maybe, in the end, life is always defined not by what we lost but what we let in.

Appendix: The Three 'P's

There are nine standards of care covered by the National Bereavement Care Pathway (NBCP). Marc Harder, NBCP UK Project Lead at Sands, explains how they break down into three subcategories, one covering the needs of bereaved parents, one covering the needs of healthcare professionals and one making sure processes are streamlined so that a bereaved family does not get a knock on the door from a cheery midwife a month after their baby has died (something that happened to a couple from the Midlands just two years ago) congratulating them and asking how baby is doing.

Marc emphasises that the NBCP is not just about stillbirth and neonatal deaths; it's about all pregnancy loss including earlier miscarriages, those choosing to end a pregnancy for medical reasons and sudden infant death. And as feedback from the handful of pilot sites which had adopted the pathway was curated, Sands went on to identify nine standards of care that all newly bereaved parents should be able to expect when their baby dies:

P FOR PARENTS

1 We want parents to have a bereavement room or bereavement suite away from happy mothers carrying a scan of a healthy baby and for those parents bereaved by miscar-

riage; and in later stages, away from parents whose baby has not been stillborn. These need to be away from the busyness of the clinic and the labour ward.

2 Give bereaved parents the opportunity to make memories. Create the space and time for them to do so. There should be cold cots, memory boxes, perhaps a photographer who can come in to take sensitive pictures of the family with their baby, or healthcare professionals who've been trained to do that.

3 We need to make sure healthcare professionals are well informed so they can give bereaved parents the opportunity to make good choices. Parents might be asked if they want their baby to have a post-mortem, for example, but parents often talk about the fog of their grief and of feeling they were in no position to make any decision. We need to think about how we give parents the chance to make good decisions and even how we give them a second chance to make the decisions that need to be made by giving them time and coming back in 24 hours to ask again. Parents need information in order to make a sound choice they won't regret later on.

P FOR PROFESSIONALS

1 Bereavement training around baby loss. We know this has improved, but there are still many trusts that don't offer this training for healthcare professionals; in fact, we've run workshops where staff have taken a day of annual leave in order to attend and even paid for the workshop themselves.

Knowing how to care for a newly bereaved parent needs to be part of their toolkit. Not just in maternity but in earlier pregnancy loss too. They need to know how to communicate well.

2 Bereavement Lead for Pregnancy Loss in each trust. This should be someone who takes responsibility for ensuring bereavement training takes place and that there is a continuity of care for bereaved parents and a consistency of approach between all the departments that may be involved with the family.

3 Support and resources for healthcare staff; not only with the specialist training in bereavement care following pregnancy loss and the death of a baby, but support for them too. We know healthcare professionals invest a tremendous amount of professional, personal and emotional energy in bereaved families at the time they need it most and if you are giving out that much support, you need to be able to talk to someone about how you have been affected by those losses.

P FOR PROCESSES

1 Parent-led bereavement care plan. This not only explains the story but also what is going to happen next. This is particularly important when bereaved parents return back into the community after leaving hospital and, of course, if there is a subsequent pregnancy. This also means parents don't have to keep telling their story again and again.

2 Bereavement Signal System. This can be as simple as a teardrop sticker on Mum's medical notes so as soon as a midwife or other health professional picks those notes up, they know, before they've even opened the front page, that there's been a bereavement. Some trusts now use a butterfly sticker which they put on the cot of a surviving twin so the healthcare professionals walking into that room know at a glance the other twin has died.

3 Having a referral process in place. The focus of the NBCP is about bereavement care during that loss, but healthcare professionals need to know where they can refer parents once they leave hospital and know what those referral processes are. Some parents will have amazing bereavement care at the hospital but that can be a bit of a bubble because they then go home and there's nothing to support them.

For more on the NBCP you can visit the dedicated website: www.nbcpathway.org.uk

Health professionals and other bereavement support parties can also sign up for e-learning modules here: www.e-lfh.org.uk/programmes/national-bereavement-care-pathway/

Sands Support

Sands supports anyone affected by the death of a baby, works to improve bereavement care and funds research to save babies' lives.

General enquiries
020 7436 7940
info@sands.org.uk
www.sands.org.uk

Postal address
Sands
Victoria Charity Centre
11 Belgrave Road
London
SW1V 1RB

Support
0808 164 3332
helpline@sands.org.uk

Sands online community
www.sands.community

Sands Bereavement Support app
www.sands.org.uk/app

Acknowledgements

One of Sands' three core aims is to support anyone affected by the death of a baby, and this book would not have been written without the generosity and bravery of those very people being prepared to share their own experiences, thoughts and reflections.

In particular, our heartfelt thanks to all those bereaved parents and families whose extraordinary generosity means that they want to make sure nobody else has to go through what they have been through; whose bravery means that they want to use their own experiences to reach out and help others; and whose determination and passion make Sands the amazing and unique charity that it is.

Thanks are also due to those professionals, clinicians, researchers and Sands staff who care so deeply about the bereaved parents and families, and who want so desperately to save babies' lives.

It is a privilege to be a part of so much passion and commitment – a privilege to be a part of Sands.

Thank you to all those who made this book possible.

Dr Clea Harmer, Chief Executive of Sands

This may read like an alphabetical list of names – which it is – but everyone I am thanking here will know why. I hope you know, too, that I would have struggled to write any part of this book without your unequivocal support and encouragement. To each of you, thank you. Beverley Bailey, Gary Cook, Susan D'Arcy, Yvonne Ferrell, Andrea Gear, Harriet Griffey, Sandra Makein, Richard Mizen, Mila Muzard Clark and Declan O'Mahony.

This book would not exist at all without my literary agent, Charlie Viney, who recognised there was a story (the story of Sands) to tell and a taboo to break; and it would not be the book it became without the thoughtful insights of our editor – Julia Kellaway – who made it look easy to wade through words, words, words; many of them, inevitably, quite harrowing, and help us find a way to show the reader that there really is no feeling of loss too terrible to be faced and overcome, primarily with the help of those who have already walked the same path and the understanding of those who love us.

And talking of those who have walked this path, thank you to every parent who spoke to me and shared their story for the book. There was not a single conversation I had with any of you that did not leave me feeling humbled; in awe of your courage and compassion for others.

Finally, thank you to our publisher, Liz Gough, for commissioning the book for Yellow Kite, for sticking with it and us despite the best efforts of coronavirus to derail us all and, of course, thank you to everyone at Sands who contributed their time and expertise and trusted us collectively to put their work and legacy on to the page.

Susan Clark

References

Pages 15, 76, 97, 156 and 226
Heazell, A. E., Siassakos, D., Blencowe, H., Burden, C., Bhutta, Z. A., Cacciatore, J., Dang, N., Das, J., Flenady, V., Gold, K. J. and Mensah, O. K., 2016. 'Stillbirths: economic and psychosocial consequences', *The Lancet*, *387*(10018), pp. 604–16. Retrieved from https://www.thelancet.com/journals/lancet/article/PIIS0140-6736(15)00836-3/fulltext (accessed 14 Jul. 2020).

Page 52
Homer, C. S., Malata, A. and ten Hoope-Bender, P., 2016. 'Supporting women, families, and care providers after stillbirths', *The Lancet*, *387*(10018), pp. 516–7. Retrieved from https://www.thelancet.com/journals/lancet/article/PIIS0140-6736(15)01278-7/fulltext (accessed 14 Jul. 2020).

Page 93
Horton, R. and Samarasekera, U., 2016. 'Stillbirths: Ending an epidemic of grief', *The Lancet*, *10018*(387), pp. 515–6. Retrieved from https://www.thelancet.com/journals/lancet/article/PIIS0140-6736(15)01276-3/fulltext (accessed 14 Jul. 2020).

Index